Palgrave Studies in Medieval and Early Modern Medicine

Series Editors
Jonathan Barry
Department of History
University of Exeter
Exeter, UK

Fabrizio Bigotti
Institute for the History of Medicine
Julius Maximilian University
Würzburg, Germany

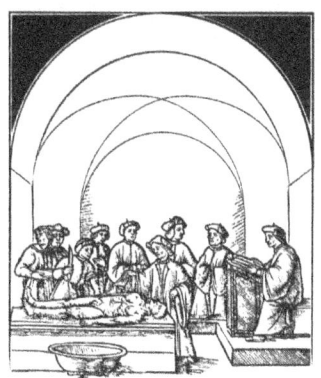

CENTRE FOR THE STUDY OF
MEDICINE AND THE BODY
IN THE RENAISSANCE

The series focuses on the intellectual tradition of western medicine as related to the philosophies, institutions, practices, and technologies that developed throughout the medieval and early modern period (500-1800). Partnered with the Centre for the Study of Medicine and the Body in the Renaissance (CSMBR), it seeks to explore the range of interactions between various conceptualisations of the body, including their import for the arts (e.g. literature, painting, music, dance, and architecture) and the way different medical traditions overlapped and borrowed from each other. The series particularly welcomes contributions from young authors. The editors will consider proposals for single monographs, as well as edited collections and translations/editions of texts, either at a standard length (70-120,000 words) or as Palgrave Pivots (up to 50,000 words).

Tommaso Ghezzani

The 'Kiss' and the Medicine of Love

A Critical Edition of Francesco Patrizi's *Il Delfino*

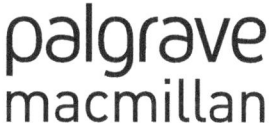

Tommaso Ghezzani
Transnational Italian Studies
Bryn Mawr College
Bryn Mawr, PA, USA

ISSN 2524-7387   ISSN 2524-7395   (electronic)
Palgrave Studies in Medieval and Early Modern Medicine
ISBN 978-3-031-75282-7   ISBN 978-3-031-75283-4   (eBook)
https://doi.org/10.1007/978-3-031-75283-4

This Palgrave Macmillan imprint is published by the registered company Springer Nature Switzerland AG
The registered company address is: Gewerbestrasse 11, 6330 Cham, Switzerland

If disposing of this product, please recycle the paper.

PREFACE

The name of Francesco Patrizi da Cherso (1529–1597) is little known today beyond the walls of universities. However, in the second half of the sixteenth century Patrizi was, like many intellectuals of the time, a prominent figure on the European stage. In Italy, he was hailed as the most authoritative Platonic philosopher of the age. He steered Renaissance Platonism into relatively unknown waters and the first university chair in Platonic philosophy was established specifically for him, first at the Studio di Ferrara and later at the Sapienza of Rome; at that time, such a position was unique within Europe.

The labels of 'Platonist' and 'professor of Philosophy' nevertheless proved somewhat restrictive for Patrizi, who preferred to present himself as an atypical intellectual, sometimes altering details of his biography to this end. For instance, in a well-known autobiographical letter of 1587, written when he was already a highly regarded professor and a courtier of the enlightened Alfonso II d'Este, duke of Ferrara, he reflects on his education but offers little to no detail concerning his specifically philosophical activity. He focuses instead on his extensive voyages at sea, which began at a very early age from his home island of Cres (at that time under Venetian rule) and took him as far afield as Greece and Spain. He also dwells on his various occupations during his career: administering villages, searching for and selling manuscripts, and publishing. The only hint of philosophical interest that emerges from the letter is a strong aversion to the Aristotelianism of the universities: a distinctive feature of

Patrizi's thought that he traces back to an underwhelming experience at the University of Padua, first as a student of medicine and later of philosophy.

Even while establishing himself as a leading intellectual at the court of Ferrara, Patrizi continued to stress the uncompromising nature of his intellectual role, in accordance with the ideological position that drove his philosophy. He held that the individual should not be removed from the practical and civic consequences of knowledge, and that true philosophy is capable of bridging the gap between *words* and *things*, functioning as an authentic, practical tool rather than empty sophistic abstraction. Patrizi's Platonism is characterised by a strong interest in the most tangible aspects of human experience, building on the most recent intellectual innovations of the century rather than the withdrawn and contemplative *pater platonicae familiae* of the Renaissance, Marsilio Ficino, who he nevertheless recognises as foundational. In addition to an interest in the more disenchanted aspects of political thought, derived from the work of Machiavelli, Patrizi also engaged in important discussions with the circle of the heterodox philosopher and natural scientist Bernardino Telesio, emphasising naturalistic dimension of the Platonic tradition. The linguistic sphere also plays a crucial role in Patrizi's thinking, reflecting vibrant contemporary interest in the arts of discourse (rhetoric and dialectic) as new tools with which to re-establish traditional knowledge.

Despite the often original and disruptive character of the Platonic thought that he brought to the everyday life of the courts and politico-cultural milieu of his time, Patrizi has largely been relegated to the conversation of specialists, above all historians of philosophy. The primary obstacle to Patrizi's diffusion across a broader range of disciplinary contexts and among a more varied public—as is the case with other authors of the period, such as Giordano Bruno or Tommaso Campanella—is undoubtedly the status of his works, which are hardly accessible to non-specialists. Almost all of Patrizi's writings survive in a philologically complex condition, with no translations or commentary to make them more approachable. I have therefore decided to take a first step towards bridging this historiographical gap, beginning with a rather peculiar work by Patrizi, his short dialogue *Delfino overo del Bacio* (*Delfino, or the Kiss*), written around 1555. For the first time, this edition presents not only an English translation of the *Delfino*, but also the first detailed commentary on the text, which is enhanced with exegetical notes. However, the primary motivation behind this volume is to provide, again for the first time, a critical and philologically accurate edition of the original Italian text. The only previous critical edition of this work exists in a single manuscript dating from 1975 and presents significant issues, with numerous errors that often compromise the meaning of Patrizi's discourse (on this subject see the *Critical note*). My aim has therefore been to provide a text that is accurate, but also easily accessible. To this end, the introductory essay presented here reinforces and completes the exegetical notes, seeking not only to contextualise Patrizi's text but also to provide an understanding of its fundamental contextual framework, that of the philosophy and medical-physiological theories of Ficino, which are nevertheless significantly reformulated in the *Delfino*.

Patrizi conceived this juvenile work to be appealing and accessible to the multifaceted public of the elegant courts and Venetian academic circles of his time. It has the advantage of offering a first glimpse into the disruptive character of his Platonism within the light-hearted dialogical frame of a pleasant and sometimes poetic conversation. Taking as his pretext a problem that at that time was, perhaps like today, considered particularly current—the pleasure provoked by a passionate kiss—Patrizi offers sharp insight into many of the foremost sources and elements of contemporary philosophy and *amorous medicine* of Platonic descent. It is especially noteworthy that Patrizi had initially trained as a physician. Beginning from a seemingly frivolous subject matter, he presents to a suitably young and impatient interlocutor, Angelo Delfino, a series of complex theories on the descent of the soul through the celestial spheres, the complex physiological mechanisms that regulate the movement of blood and *spiritus*, and the principles that underpin falling in love, drawing on both spiritual and medical/anatomical traditions.

Patrizi's principal source is undoubtedly one of the most successful texts of the fifteenth and sixteenth centuries, Ficino's *On the Nature of Love* (*El libro dell'amore*), a self-translation of his commentary on Plato's *Symposium*. Ficino, who like Patrizi first trained as a physician, presents a highly influential discussion of the physiology of erotic illness, above all in the seventh chapter of his work, which delivers a strong condemnation of the carnal aspects of amorous experience. Ficino presents the exchange of glances between lover and beloved as the root cause which, via the contamination of visual rays—that is, the transmission of blood between one body and another—triggers the mechanism of amorous illness. This is a disease in every sense of the word. Following the contamination of blood, physical turmoil passes from the body to the mind, and from the mind once again to the body; the two are considered closely linked. The examples of the madness that characterises the lovesick person and his weakened physical state are extremely eloquent. The young Patrizi clearly and somewhat precociously senses the limits of Ficino's approach, and while copies entire sections of the medical treatise of *On the Nature of Love*, sometimes word for word, he altogether alters their meaning. In the *Delfino*, the exchange of organic substance between lover and beloved does not provoke illness: on the contrary, the (physical and mental) pleasure that derives from it, culminating in the passionate tongue kiss, is if anything healthy and natural. The Platonic model must therefore come to terms with the romantic realities of the world. Patrizi endows it with a new and strong emphasis on the complex and multiple facets of the human being, comprised of soul and body, that can be read on a metaphysical level but also in relation to physiology and medicine.

As this project reaches its conclusion, I cannot fail to thank all those who have contributed to its fruition. I am especially grateful to Lina Bolzoni, whose conversations concerning Patrizi's amorous and poetic writings first prompted me to consider preparing an amended critical edition of this work, which clearly deserves to circulate in the correct textual form. Heartfelt thanks are also due to Nicola Panichi, whose guidance is invariably indispensable; to Andrea Carlino and Amneris Roselli, for having discussed these pages in great detail; to Martina de Laurentiis for generously sharing her expertise in medieval and humanistic philology. Finally, my particular gratitude goes to Jonathan Barry and Fabrizio Bigotti, who welcomed this project into their series. In particular, I am grateful to Fabrizio for allowing me to join the Centre for the Study of Medicine and the Body in the Renaissance (CSMBR), where, as a Santorio Fellow, I have come to know a stimulating and vibrant research community, characterised by excellent scholars and exemplary human beings.

New York   Tommaso Ghezzani
April 2024

CONTENTS

Timeline of Patrizi's Life and Principal Works

1529   Born in Cres, at that time under Venetian rule.
1542   Studies at Venice.
1544–1545   Studies at Ingolstadt.
1547–1554   Studies at University of Padua and becomes involved in various Venetian intellectual circles.
1553   Publishes first collection of philosophical essays: *La città felice. Dialogo dell'honore, il Barignano. Discorso della diversità de' furori poetici. Lettura sopra il sonetto del Petrarca*. La gola, e'l sonno e l'ociose piume (Venice).
1554–1557   Employed as secretary and administrator by notable Venetians.
c. 1555   Drafts *Il Delfino overo del Bacio*.
1557   Publishes *L'Eridano* (Ferrara), a laudatory poem dedicated to the Este family.
1557–1559   Member of the Accademia Veneziana (Accademia della Fama).
1558   Drafts *Il Badoaro*, a laudatory poem dedicated to Federico Badoer, the founder of the Accademia della Fama.
1560   Publishes *Della Historia* (Venice), a collection of dialogues, and a *Discorso* on the *Rime* of Luca Contile (Venice).

1560–1568	Employed as secretary and administrator by notable Venetians in Cyprus; refines ability in Greek, hunts for manuscripts.
1562	Publishes *Della Retorica* (Venice), a collection of dialogues.
1568–1573	Sells manuscripts in Spain; establishes (short-lived) publishing house *l'Elefanta*; exchange with the circle of Bernardino Telesio.
1571	Publishes the first part of *Discussiones Peripateticae* (Venice).
1575	Employed at the court of Phillip II in Madrid, where he adds to the holdings of the library of El Escorial and serves as a military consultant.
1577	Employed in Modena as a tutor the poet Tarquinia Molza; drafts the incomplete *Amorosa filosofia*.
1578–1592	Employed in Ferrara at the court of Alfonso II d'Este, serving as advisor to the duke and the very first professor of Platonic philosophy.
1581	Publishes complete edition of *Discussiones Peripateticae* (Basel).
1585	Publishes his *Parere* in defence of Ariosto's *Orlando furioso*.
1586	Drafts the first two decades of his incomplete *Poetica*, the *Deca Istoriale* (Ferrara) and *Deca Disputata* (Ferrara).
1587	Drafts the third, fourth, and fifth decades of the *Poetica*, the *Deca Ammirabile*, *Deca Plastica*, and *Deca Dogmatica Universale*; begins drafting the sixth decade, the *Deca Sacra*.
1588	Completes *Deca Sacra* and drafts the last decade before the work is interrupted, the *Deca Semisacra*.
1591	Publishes *Nova de universis philosophia* (Ferrara).
1592–1597	Employed in Rome at the Sapienza as the city's first university professor of Platonic philosophy.
1592–1594	Inquisition investigates *Nova de universis philosophia*, which is added to the Index *donec corrigatur*.
1597	Dies in Rome.

LIST OF FIGURES

Cures for Memory and Cures for the Soul: Amorous *Wounds* and Carnality Between Marsilio Ficino and Francesco Patrizi

From antiquity to the modern age, the theme of the wound has spanned the most disparate contexts, including literature, medical science, and philosophy.[1] One of the foremost interpretations of the wound is found within the semantics of love: an interpretation so influential that even today it remains part of our shared language. This connection between different disciplines comes to the fore in the first paradigmatic example of Marsilio Ficino's (1433–1499) thought, the *Commentary on Plato's Symposium* (*Commentarium in Convivium Platonis*, 1469), which disseminated his philosophy not only among philosophers but also a broader intellectual audience (literati, visual artists, etc.), especially in its

---

[1] For a spotlight on this subject in the early modern context, see Andrea Torre, *Scritture ferite. Innesti, doppiaggi e correzioni nella letteratura rinascimentale* (Venice: Marsilio, 2019).

This introductory essay presents a significantly expanded version of my Italian publication: Tommaso Ghezzani, 'Medicamenti della memoria e medicamenti dell'anima: *ferita* amorosa e carnalità tra Marsilio Ficino e Francesco Patrizi,' *Bruniana & Campanelliana*, 29 (2023).

vernacular version, *On the Nature of Love* (*El libro dell'amore*).[2] The work is composed of seven orations that mirror the structure of Plato's *Symposium*. It is in the seventh oration, which deals with amorous illness, that the interweaving of philosophical speculation and medical-physiological investigation reaches its peak. Almost a century later, Francesco Patrizi da Cherso (1529–1597) upended Ficino's paradigm in a juvenile dialogue, *Delfino, or the Kiss* (*Delfino overo del Bacio*, c. 1555), which would only be published for the first time in 1975.[3] By echoing the earlier

---

[2] For a framework of the various themes of this text see Sebastiano Gentile, '*Commentarium in Convivium de amore / El libro dell'Amore* di Marsilio Ficino' in *Letteratura italiana. Le opere, vol. 2*, edited by Alberto Asor Rosa (Milan: Einaudi, 1992): 743–767, and Maria Christine Leitgeb, *Amore e magia. La nascita di Eros e il* De amore *di Ficino* (Lucca: Cahiers Accademia, 2006). Also useful is Eugenio Canone, 'Il «senso» nei trattati d'amore: Ficino e la fortuna del modello platonico nel Cinquecento' in *Sensus-Sensatio. VIII Colloquio internazionale del Lessico Intellettuale Europeo*, edited by Massimo L. Bianchi (Florence: Olschki, 1996): 177–198.

[3] For general background on Patrizi see above all Margherita Palumbo, 'Patrizi, Francesco' in *Dizionario biografico degli italiani, vol. 81* (Rome: Istituto dell'Enciclopedia italiana, 2014), including for further bibliography, and Elisabetta Scapparone, 'Patrizi, Francesco' in *Il Contributo italiano alla storia del Pensiero – Filosofia* (Rome: Istituto dell'Enciclopedia Italiana, 2012). Other helpful contributions include: Paul O. Kristeller, *Eight Philosophers of the Italian Renaissance* (Stanford-California: Stanford University Press, 1964), 110–126; Maria Muccillo, 'La dissoluzione del paradigma aristotelico' in *Le filosofie del Rinascimento*, edited by Cesare Vasoli (Milan: B. Mondadori, 2002): 506–533; Ead., 'Philosophy and Orthodoxy: Valuation and Devaluation of the Platonic Tradition in the Late Renaissance' in *Transforming Topoi: The Exigencies and Impositions of Tradition*, edited by A.J. Johnston et al. (Göttingen: V&R, 2018): 89–118. Also worthy of consideration are the collected volumes edited by Patrizia Castelli, *Francesco Patrizi. Filosofo platonico nel crepuscolo del Rinascimento* (Florence: Olschki, 2002), and Tomáš Nejeschleba and Paul R. Blum, *Francesco Patrizi. Philosopher of the Renaissance* (Olomouc: Centre for Renaissance Texts, 2014). For an initial overview of the state of research into Patrizi, see Sandra Plastina, 'La figura e l'opera di Francesco Patrizi da Cherso nella critica più recente,' *Bruniana & Campanelliana*, 3 (1997): 335–344, and Ovanes Akopyan, 'Francesco Patrizi da Cherso (1529–1597): New Perspectives on a Renaissance Philosopher,' *Intellectual History Review*, 29 (2019): 541–543 (the introduction to a special issue on Patrizi of the *Intellectual History Review*: *Francesco Patrizi da Cherso: Ancient Wisdom, Natural Philosophy and Poetics in the Late Renaissance*). For the differences between Patrizi and Ficino, see in particular Maria Muccillo, 'Marsilio Ficino e Francesco Patrizi da Cherso' in *Marsilio Ficino e il ritorno di Platone. Studi e documenti, vol. 2*, edited by Gian Carlo Garfagnini (Florence: Olschki 1986): 615–679; Jacomien Prins, *Echoes of an Invisible World. Marsilio Ficino and Francesco Patrizi on Cosmic Order and Music Theory* (Leiden-Boston: Brill, 2014); Tommaso Ghezzani, *Il Platonico innamorato. Poesia, Amore, Magia in Francesco Patrizi da Cherso* (Florence: Olschki, 2023). For the dating of the *Delfino* I refer to the analysis of Danilo Aguzzi Barbagli, 'Un contributo di Francesco Patrizi da Cherso alle dottrine rinascimentali sull'amore,' *Yearbook of Italian*

text, sometimes *verbatim*, Patrizi overturns Ficino's condemnation of carnal love, instead using the same sources and medical and physiological thought to emphasise the importance of corporeality in human experience.

Although the gap between the peculiar Platonism of Patrizi and that of Ficino has been the subject of much scholarship, Patrizi's juvenile reworking of the medical-physiological theme has not received the attention it deserves; the same is true of the specifically physiological reflections in Ficino's *On the Nature of Love*. This essay focuses on the medical discussion in Ficino's text and its radical resumption and re-reading in the *Delfino*. One of the idiosyncrasies of Ficino's thought is his attention to the grey area that is the point of connection between body and soul, between physicality and rationality. Patrizi takes this approach to its extreme consequences, as may also be observed in his more mature writings on the philosophy of love.[4] The continuity between the imaginative faculties of the human soul, physicality, and pure rationality is thus strongly reinforced. In Patrizi's drastic re-reading, carnality and the body

---

Studies, 2 (1972): 19–50, and, above all, Lina Bolzoni, 'A proposito di una recente edizione di inediti patriziani,' *Rinascimento*, 16 (1976): 133–156, who, in addition to providing an indispensable tool for confronting the many errors present in the edition of the text prepared by Aguzzi Barbagli (Francesco Patrizi, 'Il Delfino overo del Bacio' in *Lettere e opuscoli inediti* edited by Danilo Aguzzi Barbagli (Florence: Istituto Nazionale di Studi sul Rinascimento, 1975): 135–164), highlights the same scholar's unexplained change of opinion. In the aforementioned article, Aguzzi Barbagli dates the text to the 1550s, which Bolzoni considers the most likely hypothesis; however, in the introduction to the *Lettere ed opuscoli inediti*, he situates it in the 1570s, without any detailed justification (see. ibid, xxiii). The most recent edition of the text, a French translation, is based on Aguzzi Barbagli's critical edition and inherits many of its errors; the translator amends only nine of a much greater number (see Francesco Patrizi, *Du baiser*, edited by Sylvie Laurens Aubry (Paris: Les Belles Lettres, 2002): 89–90). For further detail on these points, see the *Critical Note*.

[4] The most significant expression of this aspect of Ficino's thought is Marsilio Ficino, *Three Books on Life* (Arizona: Medieval & Renaissance Texts & Studies – The Renaissance Society of America, 1998). Patrizi's other two writings on the philosophy of love, which further develop the position advanced in the *Delfino*, are Francesco Patrizi, 'Discorso di M. Francesco Patritio,' in Luca Contile, *Le rime di Messer Luca Contile, divise in tre parti, con discorsi, et argomenti di M. Francesco Patritio, et M. Antonio Borghesi. Nuovamente stampate. Con le sei Canzoni dette le* Sei Sorelle di Marte (Venice: F. Sansovino, 1560): 14r–25v, and Francesco Patrizi, *L'amorosa filosofia*, edited by John C. Nelson (Florence: Le Monnier, 1963). There is also an English edition of the latter work: Id., *The Philosophy of Love*, edited by D. Pastina and J. W. Crayton (Philadelphia: Xlibris, 2003).

no longer constitute an obstacle to correct ascent of the Platonic *scala amoris* but, if used judiciously, lead towards the full realisation of human nature. Prompted by new cultural demands and new social contexts, Platonism enters into dialogue with the *natural* world.

The Danger of Carnality in Ficino's 'On the Nature of Love'

Even today, we may say that 'man and his attitudes constitute the point of departure of Ficino's philosophy. In this fact we must look for the secret of his historical, philosophical, and human influence and significance'.[5] Such a claim also implies important theoretical nuances within Ficino's philosophical system. It is no coincidence that the problem of the human soul's *intermediary* nature often takes centre stage, precisely on account of the attention Ficino seeks to dedicate to the distinguishing features of the human being. His conception is one of a complex amalgamation, capable of looking towards both transcendency and materiality. Such a nature is clearly emblemised by the image Ficino proposes in the culmination of his philosophical study, the *Platonic Theology* (*Theologia platonica*) (IX-7): when a weight is thrown in the air, its weight and lightness participate in equal measure whether it is rising or falling, and in the same way the human soul participates in both eternity and the temporal. The soul's dual outlook evidently has implications for the various aspects that characterise it: the phenomenon of love, of course, but also the epistemological process related to it. *Memory* plays a fundamental role in this process; but it is first necessary to specify the paradigm of memory to which Ficino refers.

In a certain sense, we may speak of a combination of two fundamental epistemological paradigms: that of Plato, which clearly dominates, and that of Aristotle. The first is rooted in a clearly delineated model of memory as a *divine* experience, codified through the archaic poetic-religious tradition, in which memory is a divine gift by which the inspired poet-priest could come to the knowledge of past and/or transcendent truths. In this sense, remembering was equivalent to knowledge of truth, laying the groundwork for what would become Platonic *anamnesis:* the recollection of innate knowledge lying dormant within the soul. The

---

[5] Paul O. Kristeller, *The Philosophy of Marsilio Ficino* (Gloucester: P. Smith, 1964): 401.

second paradigm, meanwhile, is founded on a model of memory as a *physical-individual* experience whose physiological and psychological mechanisms could be investigated. Where the former is grounded in poets such as Hesiod, or by Orphic and Pythagorean mysteries, the latter is first and foremost grounded in medical study and the activity of rhetoricians who devised fully-fledged empirical systems in order to commit long discourses to memory, the so-called *art of memory*. Broadly speaking, the former is resumed by Platonic epistemology and the latter by Aristotelian epistemology.[6]

In emphasising certain patterns that are already present in Platonic and neo-Platonic thought, Ficino dedicates significant attention to the *perceptible* aspect of the anamnestic process. As *On the Nature of Love* makes strikingly clear, although truth is already innately present within the soul, and that which is material cannot touch it directly, the stimulus of perceptible experience is nevertheless crucial in order to initiate anamnesis, the rediscovery of that latent truth. The inferior imaginative faculty (*imaginatio* (imagination), understood as the organ that reproduces perceptible experience) and superior imaginative faculty (*phantasia* (fantasy), understood as an organ that actively reimagines) assume a fundamental role in this process. The innatist principle evidently applies to both, as to the superior and immaterial intellectual faculties of the soul; thinking through *mental images* thus constitutes a progressive recovery of images that are already present, yet dormant.[7] Sensible experience then, when correctly

---

[6] On the first model see Jean Pierre Vernant, *Myth and Thought among the Greeks* (London – Bonston – Melbourne – Henley: Routledge & Kegan, 1983): 75–105. For an introduction to the second, see the classic Frances A. Yates, *The Art of Memory* (Chicago – London: University of Chicago Press, 1966): 1–26. For philosophical reworkings of these models see above all Maria Michela Sassi, 'The Greek Philosophers on How to Memorise—And Learn' in *Greek Memories. Theories and Practices*, edited by Luca Castagnoli and Paola Ceccarelli (Cambridge: Cambridge University Press, 2019): 343–361.

[7] For general discussions of the imagination in the Renaissance, see Ioan P. Couliano, *Eros and Magic in the Renaissance* (Chicago – London: University of Chicago Press, 1987): 3–27; Francesco Piro, *Il retore interno. Immaginazione e passioni all'alba della età moderna* (Naples: La Città del Sole, 1999); Nicola Panichi's commentary in his edition of Michel de Montaigne, *De la force de l'imagination. Essais, I, 21* (Paris: Classiques Garnier, 2021): 11–61; and Francesco Molinarolo's commentary in his edition of Giovanni Francesco Pico della Mirandola, *L'immaginazione* (Pisa: Edizioni della Normale – Istituto Nazionale di Studi sul Rinascimento, 2022): 7–168. On Ficino in particular, see Eugenio Garin, '*Phantasia* e *Imaginatio* fra Marsilio Ficino e Pietro Pomponazzi' in *Phantasia-Imaginatio. V Colloquio internazionale del Lessico Intellettuale Europeo*, edited by Marta Fattori and Massimo L. Bianchi (Rome: Edizioni dell'Ateneo, 1988): 3–20;

understood and accumulated, offers human beings the opportunity to rediscover their own rational-transcendent essence.

Drawing in particular on the Platonic blueprint of the *Phaedrus*, Ficino specifies which perceptible element is capable of initiating anamnesis— after all, *On the Nature of Love* is a commentary that summarises not only the claims of the *Symposium* but Plato's broader thought on love. The element in question is perceptible beauty, the prime mover of amorous desire; anamnesis and falling in love ultimately coincide.[8] Nevertheless, while Plato considers beauty to be one Idea among many, distinguished by its greater capacity for being perceived in the sensible world, in *On the Nature of Love* beauty becomes a property that belongs to all creation. It is conceived as the *visible* part of the Good in all its various degrees, the essential root of all beings under the headship of God, the supreme good.[9] By defining love as a desire for the beauty that characterises the harmony of the degrees of the universe—and a desire specific to human beings—Ficino establishes a deep connection between falling in love,

---

Stefano Benassi, 'Marsilio Ficino e il potere dell'immaginazione,' *I castelli di Yale*, 2 (1997): 1–18; Nicoletta Tirinnanzi, *Umbra naturae. L'immaginazione da Ficino a Bruno* (Rome: Edizioni di Storia e Letteratura, 2000); and above all Simone Fellina, *Modelli di episteme neoplatonica nella Firenze del '400* (Florence: Olschki 2014). For a succinct overview, albeit one that is not always clear on account of the ambiguity of certain aspects of Ficino's psychology, see Kristeller, *The Philosophy of Marsilio Ficino*, 367–384.

[8] 'Now beauty, as we said, shone bright amidst these visions, and in this world below we apprehend it through the clearest of our senses, clear and resplendent. For sight is the keenest mode of perception vouchsafed us through the body; wisdom, indeed, we cannot see thereby – how passionate had been our desire for her, if she had granted us so clear an image of herself to gaze upon – nor yet any other of those beloved objects, save only beauty; for beauty alone this has been ordained, to be most manifest to sense and most lovely of them all' (Plato, *Phaedrus*, edited by R. Hackforth (Cambridge: Cambridge University Press, 1997), (250 d), 93).

[9] 'In all these, it is the inner perfection that produces the outer perfection. This is why we say that *beauty* is the flowering of *goodness*. [...] From what has been said, I think it has been shown quite clearly that there is as much difference between goodness and beauty as there is between seed and flower' (Marsilio Ficino, *On the Nature of Love: Ficino on Plato's Symposium* (London: Shepheard-Walwyn, 2016), (V-1), 55, my italics ('In tutte le cose la perfectione di dentro produce la perfectione di fuori, e quella chiamiamo *bonità*, e questa *bellezza*; per la qual cosa vogliamo la bellezza essere fiore di bonità. [...] Per le cose decte, stimo essere assai dichiarato tanta differentia essere intra la bontà e la bellezza quanta è tra 'l seme e' fiori' (Marsilio Ficino, *El libro dell'amore* (Florence: Olschki, 1987), (V-1), 76, my italics)).

knowledge, and memory, the latter understood both in the specific sense of a faculty of the human soul and in terms of anamnesis.[10]

Where love is righteous and virtuous, vision of the beloved's perceptible beauty acts upon the imaginative fabric of the lover, *affecting* it deeply enough to allow a glimpse of the innate ideal image, the herald of the transcendent. Ficino has no compunction about turning to the semantic field of violence in order to describe this experience, explaining that beauty 'is called *calos* or incitement, because it greatly incites the soul. *Calos* is from the verb *caleo*, meaning "I incite", and *calos* in Greek means *beauty* in Latin'.[11] This, as we shall see, is not merely a metaphor, but literally describes the physicality of this first phase of falling in love, which is common to virtuous love and bestial love. The passage recalls the *Phaedrus*, where in the myth of the soul as a winged chariot the dazzling beauty of the beloved is translated into the violent *blow* dealt to the horses by the charioteer: 'At that sight the driver's memory goes back to that form of Beauty [...]; then in awe and reverence he falls upon his back, and therewith is compelled to pull the reins so violently that he brings both steeds down on their haunches', and, faced with the insistence of the black horse, or rather the element of the soul that desires to approach the beloved, 'he driver, with resentment even stronger than before, like a racer recoiling from the starting-rope, jerks back the bit [χαλινόν] in the mouth of the wanton horse with an even stronger pull, bespatters his railing tongue and his jaws with blood, and forcing him down on legs and haunches delivers him over to anguish'.[12] The violent 'provocation' ('*callos*') of beauty, which in Plato is characterised by real

[10] 'And when we say Love, understand Love to be the desire for beauty' (Ficino, *On the Nature of Love*, I-4), 11 ('Quando noi diciamo amore, intendete desiderio di bellezza' (Ficino, *El libro dell'amore* (I-4), 15)). It is clear that Ficino interprets the myth of the two halves of the human being as referring to the two *lights* of the human soul: the component that is intellectual and divine and component that is rational and human. The reunification of these two halves is the reascension, or memory, of the intellectual light, which has been stifled by the dominance of its human counterpart. This memory is in the first instance triggered by sensible beauty; see Ficino, *On the Nature of Love*, (IV-5), 48; *El libro dell'amore*, (IV-5), 67. See also, specifically on how the lover falls in love with the beloved, *On the Nature of Love*, (V-5), 65–66; *El libro dell'amore*, (V-5), 88–89.

[11] *On the Nature of Love*, (V-2), 55. *El libro dell'amore*, (V-2), 79: 'perché molto provoca l'animo si chiama "callos", cioè provocatione, da un verbo che dice "caleo", che vuol dire provoco, e "callos" in greco significa in latino bellezza'. As we shall see, the images used to denote the amorous illness are even stronger.

[12] Plato, *Phaedrus*, (254b–e), 104.

scars left upon the soul by the bridle (ʻχαλινός'), assumes the same image in the *Gorgias*—here in a broader context, but one nevertheless related to love—with the wicked soul displaying 'a mass of weals and scars imprinted on it by the various acts of perjury and wrong-doing of which the man has been guilty'.[13] In this case, the marks are emblematic of vice, rather than the virtuous, rational control of passionate instincts described in the *Phaedrus*; yet the idea of the scarred soul, as we shall see, will be reprised in similar terms in order to denote the marks left by bestial love upon the *spiritual* canvas, and thus upon memory. The two Platonic loci are united in Ficino's thought, in part following Porphyry's reading of the *Gorgias* (*Ad Gaurum* VI, 6–11, and IX, 3; and *De abstinentia* II, 42).[14]

In order to explain the physiological process that underpins this first phase of the erotic-anamnestic process, Ficino turns to the concepts of *ethereal body* and *spiritus*, whose respective functions are not always clear in his writing.[15] The purpose of both is to establish a *medium* between immaterial soul and material body. The first is formed from the ether of the superlunar world; the second derives from the vapour of the blood and is the fundamental means by which the soul exercises its inferior faculties, those of a nutritive and imaginative nature (Fig. 1.1).

[13] Plato, *Gorgias*, edited by W. Hamilton (Baltimore – Maryland: Penguin, 1960), (524e), 144.

[14] See Anna Corrias, 'Imagination and Memory in Marsilio Ficino's Theory of the Vehicles of the Soul,' *The International Journal of the Platonic Tradition*, 6 (2012): 81–114, especially 93–94.

[15] During the Renaissance, the two concepts were often confused with the Neoplatonic ethereal body and other religious and medical beliefs. See in particular Daniel Pickering Walker, 'The Astral Body in Renaissance Medicine,' *Journal of the Warburg and Courtauld Institutes*, 21 (1958): 119–133; Id., *Spiritual and Demonic Magic. From Ficino to Campanella* (Notre Dame: University of Notre Dame Press, 1975): 3–24; Robert Klein, *Form and Meaning. Essays on the Renaissance and Modern Art* (New York: Viking Press, 1979): 62–85; Eugenio Garin, 'Relazione introduttiva' in *Spiritus. IV Colloquio internazionale del Lessico Intellettuale Europeo*, edited by Marta Fattori and Massimo L. Bianchi (Rome: Edizioni dell'Ateneo, 1984): 3–14; Daniel Pickering Walker, 'Medical Spirits and God and the Soul' in *Spiritus*: 218–243; Couliano, *Eros and Magic in the Renaissance*, 3–27; and Corrias, *Imagination and Memory in Marsilio Ficino's Theory of the Vehicles of the Soul*, who clearly demonstrates how, in some cases, Ficino further divides the ethereal body into two constituent parts of differing purity. As many scholars have observed, and among the first Kristeller (see Kristeller, *The Philosophy of Marsilio Ficino*, 371–374), the ethereal body and aerial body are distinct concepts, even though Ficino himself often presents them ambiguously and it is often unclear how the psychological functions are divided between them.

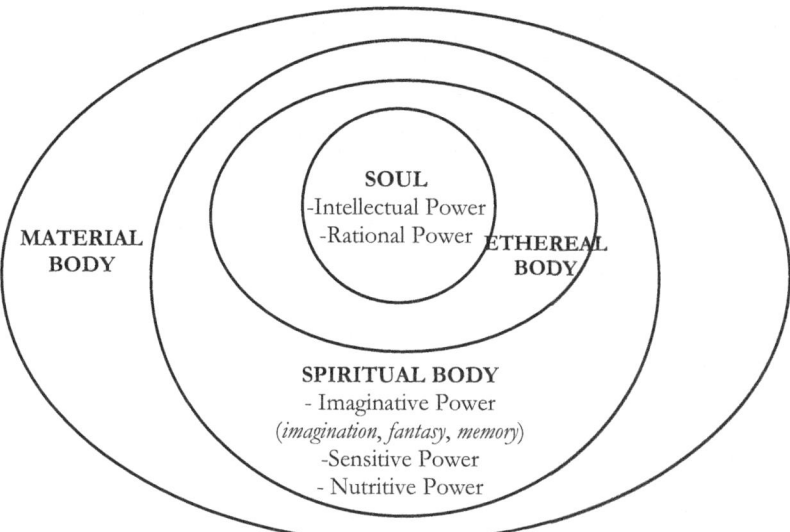

Fig. 1.1   Diagram of the human being

In his works, Ficino dedicates significant attention to the *spiritus*, which—like the *fantasy* of which it is an instrument—is a hybrid and elusive concept. Just as fantasy mediates between particular perception and universal intellection, the *spiritus* is situated between soul and body, serving as a bridge between the two, and it may thus entail both physiological and psychological questions.[16] The concept of *spiritus* is most closely dissected in *De vita libris tres* (1489), which places medical prescriptions, philosophical thought, and magical practices in dialogue. Here, the *spiritus* is defined (though in reality this is only one of multiple definitions in the course of the work) as:

> a vapor of blood – pure, subtle, hot, and clear. After being generated by the heat of the heart out of the more subtle blood, it flies to the brain; and there the soul uses it continually for the exercise of the interior as well as the exterior senses. This is why the blood subserves the spirit; the spirit, the senses; and finally, the senses, reason. Now the blood is made by that natural power which flourishes in the liver and the stomach. The lightest

[16] See Garin, '*Phantasia e Imaginatio*,' 5.

part of the blood flows into the fountain of the heart, where flourishes the vital power. The spirits generated from this ascend to the citadels of the brain and (as I might say) of Pallas.[17]

The journey of the *spiritus* begins from the heart, where blood (generated by the stomach and liver) is warmed before rising into the brain; in this regard, Ficino follows the traditions associated with Aristotle and Galen. The union between sensitive-imaginative experience, made possible through the movement of the *spiritus* to the brain, and rational experience is thus emphasised, establishing a strong connection between bodily and mental health. In *On the Nature of Love*, Ficino offers a briefer analysis, which is nevertheless useful on account of the epistemological digression, summarised above, that accompanies it:

> Within us there are undoubtedly three things: soul, spirit, and body. Soul and body are quite different by nature, and they are united by means of spirit, which is a kind of very fine bright vapour produced by the warmth of the heart from the finest parts of the blood. And being spread from here throughout all the limbs, it receives the power of the soul and conveys it to the body. Through the instruments of the senses it also receives the images of external bodies, which cannot inhere in the soul because incorporeal substance, which excels bodies, cannot be shaped by them through the receiving of images; but the soul, being present to spirit in every part, can readily see the images of bodies reflected in spirit, as in a mirror, and by these images she judges the bodies. And the followers of Plato call this cognition sensory perception. While the soul looks at them, she conceives, through her own power, images that are similar to them but much purer. The images conceived here are preserved by memory. It is by them that the eye of intellect is frequently prompted to reflect upon the universal Ideas of all things, which it holds within itself.[18]

[17] Ficino, *Three Books on Life*, (I-2), 111 ('vapor quidam sanguinis purus, subtilis, calidus et lucidus definitur. Atque ab ipso cordis calore ex subtiliori sanguine procreatus volat ad cerebrum; ibique animus ipso ad sensus tam interiores quam exteriores exercendos assidue utitur. Quamobrem sanguis spiritui servit, spiritus sensibus, sensus denique rationi. Sanguis autem a virtute naturali, quae in iecore stomachoque viget, efficitur. Tenuissima sanguinis pars fluit in cordis fontem, ubi vitalis viget virtus. Inde creati spiritus cerebri et (ut ita dixerim) Palladis arces ascendunt', ibid., 110).

[18] Ficino, *On the Nature of Love*, (VI-6), 90–91 (*El libro dell'amore*, (VI-6), 123–124: 'Tre cose sanza dubio sono in noi: anima, spirito e corpo; l'anima e 'l corpo sono di natura molto diversa: congiungonsi insieme per mezzo dello spirito, el quale è un certo vapore, sottilissimo e lucidissimo, generato pe 'l caldo del cuore della più sottile parte del

Nevertheless, in some passages of the text it appears that the higher imaginative functions are entrusted to the ethereal body and not the *spiritus*.[19] The latter returns to prominence in the seventh oration, where it is discussed in relation to bestial love.

Within the discussion of virtuous love, *anamnesis*—initiated by the *blow* exerted by beauty, derived from the sight of the body of the beloved—is presented in relation to the ethereal body, with which the soul is invested at the moment it descends to earth from the heavens and becomes incarnate. This substance is *formed* through the influence of a specific planet depending on the temporal moment at which the process occurs.[20] This astrological influence, whereby the ethereal body is shaped according to a particular planetary *form*, has consequences not only for a person's nature, but also for the appearance the material body will ultimately take and the specific way in which the soul will perceive

sangue, e di qui essendo sparso per tutti e membri, piglia le virtù dell'anima, e quelle comunica al corpo. Piglia ancora per gli instrumenti de' sensi le imagine de' corpi di fuori, le quale imagine non si possono appiccare nell'anima, però che la sustantia incorporea, che è più excellente ch'e corpi, non può essere formata da·lloro per la receptione delle imagine, ma l'anima, essendo presente allo spirito in ogni parte, agevolmente vede le imagine de' corpi come in uno specchio in essi rilucenti, e per quelle giudica e corpi, e tale cognitione è senso da' platonici chiamata. E in mentre ch'ella riguarda, per sua virtù in sé concepe imagine simile a quelle, e ancora molto più pure, e tale conceptione si chiama imaginatione e fantasia. Le imagine concepute in questo luogo conserva la memoria, e per queste è spesso incitato l'occhio dello intellecto a riguardare le idee universali di tutte le cose, le quali in sé contiene').

[19] On this subject, see also Id. 'Commentaria in Platonis "Sophistam"' in *Icastes. Marsilio Ficino's Intepretation of Plato's Sophist*, edited by Michael J. B. Allen (Berkeley: University of California Press, 1989), 272: 'You will know that the soul primarily and effectively exercises the imagination in the celestial vehicle and prepares all the sense through the whole vehicle; and through this vehicle as through a seal frequently it impresses images on the second veil; and through the second similarly it fashions the third' ('Cognoces animam primo quidem efficaciterque imaginationem in coelesti vehiculo exercere, sensumque prorsus omnem per totum vehiculum expedire; perque vehiculum hoc quasi per sigillum secundo velamini imagines frequenter imprimere; per secundum similiter tertium conformare', ibid., 273).

[20] See Ficino, *On the Nature of Love*, (VI-4), 86 et seq; *El libro dell'amore*, (VI-4), 117 et seq.

physical beauty.[21] A tripartite stratification of the *form* of beauty within the complex human psyche is thus established:

1. Universal and abstract idea of beauty (rational part of the soul)
2. Ideal visual beauty (ethereal body)
3. Particular bodily beauty (material body).

Where the bodily beauty of the beloved strikes the *spiritus*/ethereal body and *engraves* its shape in the correct way, the lover unconsciously begins to perceive, or rather remember, the ideal beauty already present within his ethereal body. This image is more true than either the beloved or the lover himself, who both descend from a common universal lineage:

> The soul [of the lover], being thus struck, recognises as here own the image of the person in front of her, an image that is almost exactly the same as the one which she has had within herself of old [...] The soul at once affixes this image onto her own inner image, imparting to it a better shape if any detail is missing from the perfect shape of the Jovian body. She then loves that re-shaped image as her own handiwork. And thus it comes about that lovers are so deceived that they judge the one they love

---

[21] *On the Nature of Love*, (VI-6), 89: 'Understand that what I say about one example applies to all the others. As a soul governed by Jupiter comes down into an earthly body, she conceives a design for crafting a person who will be comfortable to the star of Jupiter. She etches this design very precisely onto her celestial body, which is beautifully prepared to receive it. Id she finds on Earth a seed that is similarly prepared, she depicts on it a third design which closely resembles the second and the first. [...] It often happens that two souls, both under the rule of Jupiter [...] have a liking for each other on account of the similarity of their nature. [...] This is how it comes about that each person has the greatest love, not for those who are the most beautiful, but for those who are his own, by which I mean those with a similar birth-chart, even though they may not be as beautiful as many others' (*El libro dell'amore*, (VI-6), 122–123): 'Quello che io dirò nello exemplo d'uno intendete degli altri. Qualunque animo sotto lo imperio di Giove nel corpo terreno discende, concepe, nel discendere, una certa figura di fabricare uno huomo conveniente alla stella di Giove, la qual figura nel suo corpo celestiale, che è optimamente adaptato a riceverla, molto propria scolpisce. E se similmente arà trovato in terra temperato seme, ancora in quello dipigne la terza figura, molto simile alla seconda e prima. Spesso adviene che due animi saranno discesi regnante Giove, [...] amendua, per una certa similitudine di natura scambievolmente si piacciono. Vero è che [...] ciascuno maximamente ama non qualunque è bellissimo, ma ama e suoi, dico quegli che hanno avuto natività consimile, anco quando e' non fussino sì begli come molti altri').

to be more beautiful than is the case. For with the passage of time they do not see what they love in the actual image received through the senses: they see it in the image that their soul has now shaped to the likeness of their own idea.[22]

By *scraping* away the layer that covers with forgetfulness the ideal image of beauty, the lover prepares to ascend to the following stage of anamnesis, moving from a still-visual ideal beauty to a beauty that is abstract and rational, the source of true knowledge.[23] Bringing this reflection to a close, Ficino embarks on a prelude to his discussion of bestial love, which will appear in the following oration. In bestial love, the soul of the lover lacks the imagination to *scrape* away the physical contingency of the beauty of the beloved, and it therefore does not begin the ascent towards the ideal universality to which that beauty belongs. In this way, the soul 'is so enchanted by physical beauty that she commits her own beauty to oblivion; and, forgetting herself, she feverishly runs after physical beauty, the shadow of her own beauty. From this there ensues that cruel fate which Narcissus suffered and of which Orpheus sings. From this there ensues the wretched lot of mankind'.[24]

The seventh oration is devoted to discussion of the amorous illness. In Plato's *Symposium* (212c–222b), the equivalent oration describes the entry of the corrupt drunkard Alcibiades, who brings the discourse crashing back to earth following the metaphysical heights reached by Socrates and Diotima in the preceding oration. Ficino sidesteps Plato's unseemly staging, though it is evoked through his moral condemnation of

---

[22] *On the Nature of Love*, (VI-6), 89–90. *El libro dell'amore*, (VI-6), 123: 'L'animo di costui [amante], così percosso, ricognosce come cosa sua la imagine di colui [amato] che si gli fece innanzi, la quale quasi interamente è tale ab antiquo egli ha in sé medesimo, [...] e quella subitamente appicca alla sua interiore imagine, e quella riformando megliora, se parte alcuna gli manca alla perfecta forma del corpo gioviale; e dipoi essa imagine così riformata ama come sua opera propria. Di qui nasce che gli amanti sono tanto ingannati che giudicano la persona amata essere più bella ch'ella non è; imperò che in processo di tempo e' non veggono la cosa amata nella propria imagine presa pe' sensi, ma veggono quella nella imagine già formata dalla loro anima ad similitudine della loro idea'.

[23] See *On the Nature of Love*, (VI-6), 90–91; *El libro dell'amore*, (VI-6), 123–124.

[24] *On the Nature of Love*, (VI-17), 124. *El libro dell'amore*, (VI-17), 167–168; 'è tanto lusingata dalla forma corporale che manda in oblivione la propria spetie, e dimenticando sé medesima seguita ardentemente la forma del corpo, la quale è ombra della spetie dell'anima. Di qui seguita quel crudelissimo fato di Narcisso che canta Orpheo, di qui seguita la miserabile calamità degli uomini'.

the material discussed. Preceding orations have presented in the *violence* enacted upon the imaginative canvas by the sight of the lover and the impression left on the spiritual substrate in positive terms, but here we glimpse the other side of the coin. In earlier passages, the wounding of the *spiritus* is explored in terms of the progressive re-emergence of the ideal beauty that lay dormant within the ethereal body, an image of transcendent immaterial-rational beauty. Here, however, we observe that beauty's corruption. Focusing on the materiality of the *spiritus*, Ficino observes that in corrupted love, which is strictly carnal, the lover is unable to ascend to the ultimate and universal root of beauty, and instead becomes fossilised in the physical contingency of the beloved. Bestial love is moreover likened to a physical malady caused by contamination of the blood. As in the *Phaedrus*, the term *furor* carries a double meaning, referring both to that which is positive and divinely inspired (among other things) by virtuous love, and to its negative counterpart provoked by human failings. Manias are caused by disturbances to the physiological balance of the brain; similar problems within the heart are the root cause of love sicknesses.[25]

More specifically, the substantial difference between the physiological processes of virtuous love and bestial love is explained by the differing extent to which *material* perception takes root. In bestial love, the passage of material prevails over any rational reworking by the lover's soul, and the superficial physiological layer cannot be stripped away to reveal the original metaphysical root. In other words, the substance derived from perceptible experience of physical beauty is so excessively material and physiological that it prevents anamnesis of the transcendent. The memory of the lovesick person is frozen as a fixed image and, as we have seen, can never evolve into an ideal image.

The passage of material takes place through the *spiritus*, a sanguine vapour which recondenses into blood when it passes from the beloved to the lover. In this way, the amorous illness is caused by the entry of external blood into the blood of the lover. Ficino delineates the various stages of the process, beginning with the *spiritus*, which is formed in the heart before rising to the brain and exiting through the eyes.[26] This same principle underpins the transmission of viruses through the gaze:

---

[25] See *On the Nature of Love*, (VII-3), 137–138; *El libro dell'amore*, (VII-3), 187–188.

[26] See *On the Nature of Love*, (VII-4), 139; *El libro dell'amore*, (VII-4), 190.

when a diseased and a healthy person look each other in the eyes, the diseased person transmits part of their *spiritus* to their healthy counterpart through their visual rays. The diseased *spiritus* subsequently recondenses into blood within the healthy body, causing it to become sick:

> But the fact that a ray emitted through the eyes draws the spirit-vapour with it, and that this vapour draws the blood, can be understood from the following: those who stare at another's infirm and bloodshot eyes fall under the evil eye on account of the rays emanating from those infirm eyes. Thus it appears that the ray extends to the person who is watching, and the vapour of the corrupt blood accompanies the ray, and through this contamination the eye of the beholder suffers. Aristotle says that the gaze of women in their menstrual courses soils the mirror with bloody drops.[27]

More specifically, coming to the problem of the amorous illness, it is asked:

> Who, then, will be surprised to learn that if the eye is open and directed attentively at someone, it shoots the arrows of its rays at the eyes of the person who is looking at it and, together with these arrows, which are the vehicles of the spirits, it shoots that bloody vapor which we call spirit? The poisoned arrow passes through the eyes and, having been fired from the heart of the marksman, homes in on the heart of the wounded man as its own natural place of abode. Thus it wounds the heart; but it thickens on the heart's hard back and turns into blood again. This foreign blood, being alien to the nature of the stricken man, troubles his blood, which turns sour, as it were, and grows sick. From this there arises enchantment, the evil eye.[28] (Fig. 1.2)

---

[27] *On the Nature of Love*, (VII-4), 140; *El libro dell'amore*, (VII-4), 191: 'Ma che el razzo che si manda fuori per gli occhi tiri seco lo spiritale vapore, e che questo vapore tiri seco el sangue, lo possiamo di qui intendere: che quegli che fiso guardano negli occhi d'altri infermi e rossi, cascano nel male degli occhi per cagione de' razzi che vengono dagli occhi infermi, dove apparisce che el razzo si distende infino a colui che guarda, e insieme col razzo el vapore del sangue corrotto corre, per la contagione del quale l'occhio di chi vede ammala. Scrive Aristotile che le donne quando sono nel corso del sangue menstruo, spesse volte macchiano lo specchio, guardando fiso, di gocciole sanguigne'. The source is Aristotle, *De insomniis*, II, 459b.

[28] *On the Nature of Love*, (VII-4), 140–141. *El libro dell'amore*, (VII-4), 192: 'Chi si maraviglierà adunque che l'occhio aperto, e con attentione diricto inverso alcuno, saecti agli occhi di chi lo guarda le frecce de' razzi suoi, e insieme con queste frecce, che sono e carri degli spiriti, scagli quel sanguigno vapore el quale spirito chiamiamo? Di qui la

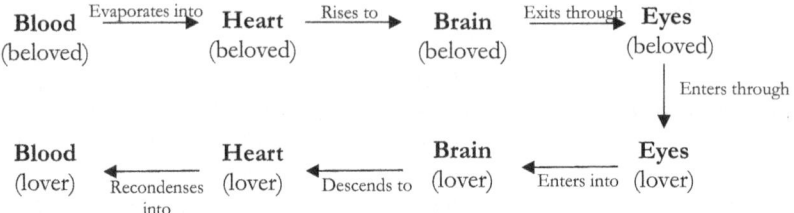

Fig. 1.2 Diagram of the blood path in falling in love

The moral and metaphysical register of previous discussions here makes way for an investigation of purely medical and physiological character, which persists for almost the entire oration. Ficino describes precisely how the visual ray of the beloved passes into the heart of the lover, wounding him and contaminating his blood. This is also the cause of the lover's crazed search for the beloved:

> Set before your eyes Phaedrus the Myrrhinusian and Lysias the Theban orator, who was enamoured of Phaedrus. [...] What happens is therefore amazing: Phaedrus blood is now in Lysias' heart! At this, each is forced to cry out. Lysias says to Phaedrus, "O Phaedrus, my heart! My dearest inwards parts!" Phaedrus says to Lysias, "O Lysias, my spirit, my blood!" Phaedrus pursues Lysias because his heart demands the return of its humour. Lysias pursues Phaedrus because the sanguine humour demands the return of its own receptacle and its own abode. But Lysias pursues Phaedrus more ardently, because the heart can live more easily without a very small droplet of its humour than can the humour without its heart. The stream needs the spring more than the spring needs the stream.[29]

venenosa freccia trapassa gli occhi, e perché l'è saettata dal cuore di chi la getta, però si getta al cuore dell'uomo ferito quasi come a regione propria a sé e naturale, quivi ferisce el cuore e nel suo dosso duro si condensa e torna in sangue. Questo sangue forestiero el quale dalla natura del ferito è alieno, turba el sangue proprio del ferito, e'l sangue turbato e quasi incertonito inferma. Di qui nasce la fascinatione, cioè mal d'occhio'.

[29] *On the Nature of Love*, (VII-4), 141–142. *El libro dell'amore*, (VII-4), 193–194: 'Ponetevi innanzi agli occhi Phedro Mirrinusio e Lysia oratore tebano di Phedro innamorato: [...] qui adviene cosa stupenda, e questa è che il sangue di Phedro già nel cuore di Lysia si truova, di qui l'uno e l'altro ad gridare è constructo. Lysia ad Phedro dice: «O cuor mio, Phedro! O mie interiori carissime!»; Phedro dice ad Lysia: «O spirito mio, o mio sangue, Lysia!». Phedro seguita Lysia perché el cuore richiede el suo humore,

The lover is consequently much more greatly attracted to the lover than vice versa, again for a purely physiological reason: the small quantity of the beloved's blood within the lover seeks to return to its place of origin with far more urgency than the beloved's heart pursues the minuscule quantity it has lost.

The result is an outright desire for revenge, which serves to explain the conflation of excessive passion and intrinsic violence that characterises bestial love. In a certain sense, the lover wishes both to possess and to destroy the beloved, as Ficino explains in relation to the risky figure of Lucretius (*De rerum natura*, IV, lines 1047–1051)[30]:

> In these lines Lucretius means that the blood of the man who has been wounded by the ray of the eyes gushes towards the man who has inflicted the wound, just as the blood of the man who has been slain with a dagger gushes towards his killer. If you are looking for the cause of this miracle, I shall explain it as follows: Hector wounds Patroclus and slays him. Patroclus turns his eyes towards Hector, who is wounding him, and as a result his thought judges that he should avenge himself. His bile is immediately kindled for revenge. The blood is immediately inflamed by the bile and, being inflamed, it gushes at once towards the wound to protect that part and also to wreak vengeance.[31]

seguita Lysia Phedro perché l'umore sanguigno richiede el proprio vaso e la propria sedia, e seguita Lysia più ardentemente Phedro, perché el cuore sanza una minima particella di suo humore più facilmente vive, che lo humore sanza el proprio cuore: el rivolo ha più bisogno del fonte che il fonte del rivulo'.

[30] On the singular Renaissance reception of Lucretius—who, although strongly heterodox, was remarkably never placed on the Index—see Valentina Prosperi, *«Di soavi licor gli orli del vaso». La fortuna di Lucrezio dall'Umanesimo alla Controriforma* (Turin: Aragno, 2004); Alison Brown, *The Return of Lucretius to Renaissance Florence* (Cambridge (MA)-London: Harvard University Press, 2010); Ada Palmer, *Reading Lucretius in the Renaissance* (Cambridge (MA)-London: Harvard University Press, 2014). On Ficino's specific use of Lucretius, see Sebastiano Gentile, 'Ficino, Epicuro e Lucrezio' in *The Rebirth of Platonic Theology. Proceedings of a conference held at The Harvard University Center for Italian Renaissance Studies (Villa I Tatti) and the Istituto Nazionale di Studi sul Rinascimento (Florence, 26–27 April 2007)*, edited by James Hankins and Fabrizio Meroi (Florence: Olschki, 2013): 119–135; Elena Nicoli, 'Ficino, Lucretius and Atomism,' *Early Science and Medicine*, 23 (2018): 330–361; Raphael Ebgi, *Voluptas. La filosofia del piacere nel giovane Marsilio Ficino (1457–1469)* (Pisa: Edizioni della Normale – Istituto Nazionale di Studi sul Rinascimento, 2019).

[31] *On the Nature of Love*, (VII-5), 143–144. *El libro dell'amore*, (VII-5), 196–197: 'Lucretio in questi versi vuole che il sangue dell'uomo, el quale dal razzo degli occhi fù ferito, corre inverso di colui che l'ha ferito, non altrimenti che il sangue di colui che fù

Just as blood influences thought through the *spiritus*, so the same is true in reverse. From a psychophysical perspective, this is the case because the blood in the heart is in direct contact with the *spiritus*, the organ of the imaginative faculty. Influencing the former necessarily implies influencing the latter and thus influencing part of thought itself, and vice versa.[32]

As a result, the contamination of blood by the entry of blood from elsewhere implies a corruption of thought. The faculties of memory and fantasy are especially compromised through this process, impeding anamnesis. It is no surprise to learn that there are physiological implications for the material body of one who is lovesick:

> And so none of you should be surprised to hear that a lover has assumed in his own body some likeness of his beloved. [...] And he therefore thinks on his beloved more fervently and more steadfastly. Thus it is no wonder that the beloved's face, being impressed on the lover's heart, is depicted in his spirit and imprinted in his blood by his spirit. [...] The parts of the body are restore by the blood, which courses from the channels of the veins. Will you therefore be surprised if blood which has been imprinted with a particular likeness sketches that likeness on the parts of the body [...]?[33]

Here, the fashionable poetic metaphor of the beloved carved within the heart of the lover is divested of its literary quality and reinterpreted from a strictly medical perspective. Through the presence of the beloved's blood within the lover, the image of the beloved is literally carved into the root of the imaginative substrate: the heart, where the *spiritus* is

---

di coltello ucciso inverso l'omicida corra. Se voi ricercate la ragione di questo miracolo io ve la chiarirò in questo modo: Hectore ferisce e uccide Patroclo; Patroclo volge gli occhi inverso Hectore che lo ferisce, onde el suo pensiero giudica doversi vendicare; subito la colera alla vendecta s'accende, dalla colera s'infiamma el sangue, el sangue infiammato subito corre alla fedita, sì per difendere quella parte, sì etiandio per vendicar'.

[32] On this notion of contagion, see also Guido Giglioni, 'Contagio e immaginazione,' *Lexicon philosophicum*, 8 (2020): 265–268.

[33] *On the Nature of Love*, (VII-8), 146. *El libro dell'amore*, (VII-8), 201–202: 'E però nessuno di voi si maravigli, se udissi alcuno innamorato avere concepto nel corpo suo alcuna similitudine della persona amata. [...] E però più forte e fermo [l'amante] cogita, sì che non è maraviglia che il volto della persona amata, scolpito nel cuore dell'amante, per tale cogitatione si dipinga nello spirito, e dallo spirito nel sangue s'imprima [...]. Rifansi e membri pe'l sangue el quale da' rivoli delle vene corre: adunque maraviglieràti tu se 'l sangue, di certa similitudine dipinto, la medesima ne' membri disegni [...]?'.

formed.[34] A passage of the sixth oration, which anticipates this discussion, develops along similar lines. Having observed that the lover's 'unremitting thought' concerning the beloved absorbs much of the *spiritus*, removing it from many of the body's other functions (such as digestion), Ficino adds that

> wherever the unremitting attention of the soul takes us, there also fly the spirits, which act as the chariot and instrument of the soul. [...] The soul of the lover is seized and carried off to the image of the beloved which is engraved in his imagination and to the actual beloved. The spirits are also drawn to the beloved, and as they fly there they are continually consumed. This is why a constant supply of pure blood is needed to replenish the spirits that are forever being consumed, for the finest and clearest parts of the blood are exhausted in replacing the spirits which never stop flying off.[35]

The mental image of the beloved dangerously absorbs a large part of the lover's *spiritus*, sapping its blood. The result is a vicious cycle in which the diseased fantasy and memory damage the body, which in turn, as a result of an imbalance of humours, further damages the thought. Excessive consumption of *spiritus* saps the blood. As a result,

> when the pure clear blood is exhausted, what is left is blood that is contaminated, thick, dry, and black. And so the body becomes dry and grows pale; and the overs become melancholic, because the melancholic humour thrives on blood that is dry, thick, and black. This humour fills the head with its vapours, makes the brain dry, and does not refrain day or night from afflicting the soul with dark, terrifying images. On account of

---

[34] On this subject, see Couliano, *Eros and Magic in the Renaissance*, 28–32, and Lina Bolzoni, *The Gallery of Memory. Literary and Iconographic Models in the Age of the Printing Press* (Toronto – Buffalo – London: University of Toronto Press, 2001): 145–162.

[35] *On the Nature of Love*, (VI-9), 98–99. *El libro dell'amore*, (VI-9), 135–136: 'dove l'assidua intentione dell'animo ci traporta, quivi volano ancora gli spiriti che sono carro e instrumento dell'anima. [...] L'animo dell'amante è rapito inverso la imagine dello amato che è nella fantasia scolpita, e inverso la persona amata. Inverso questo sono tirati ancora gli spiriti, e volando quivi continuamente si consumano, per la qual cosa è bisogno di molta materia di sangue puro a ricreare spesso gli spiriti che continuamente si risolvono, dove le più sottili e più lucide parti del sangue tutto dì si logorano, per rifare gli spiriti che continuamente volano fuori'.

protracted love, this is what happened to Lucretius, the Epicurean philosopher who, being distressed first by love and then by mad rage, took his
own life.[36]

Obsessive thought, focused on the image of the beloved, consumes
all spiritual energies and leads to the degradation of the blood, which
through imbalance becomes dense and heavy. This damaged blood causes
physical frailty and furthermore produces a vapour, though one altogether
different from the healthy *spiritus*, which rises to the brain and provokes
melancholic mania. In the theory of the four humours (blood, phlegm,
yellow bile, and black bile) on which Ficino draws, illness is generally
triggered by an excess of one in relation to the others. When black bile
is predominant it causes melancholy, which should not be understood
simply in terms of depression but rather as an altered mental state in which
moments of psychophysical stasis alternate with intense and unregulated
activity.[37] It is this that Ficino is referring to when he speaks of the ghostly
images that torture the madman. Significantly, he employs the emblematic
example of Lucretius's suicide on account of his love madness in order to
illustrate how the amorous illness can provoke one of the bleakest mental
maladies.

   In the light of these two passages, it is evident that the mental image
of the beloved, fixed within lover, prevents the lovesick individual from
thinking of anything else, exhausting the *spiritus* that is required for
other psychological and nutritive operations and upending the anamnestic
process of virtuous love. In virtuous love, the image of the beloved is
received through the senses and carved into the spiritual substrate of the
lover, from there *liberating* the ideal form of beauty concealed within

---

[36] *On the Nature of Love*, (VI-9), 99. *El libro dell'amore* (VI-9), 136–137: 'il perché
adviene che risoluto el puro chiaro sangue, rimane el sangue maculato, grosso, arido e
nero, di qui el corpo si secca e impallidisce, di qui gli amanti divengono malinconici perché
l'omore malinconico si multiplica per 'l sangue secco, grosso e nero, e questo omore co'
suoi vapori riempie il capo, disecca el celabro, e non resta dì e nocte d'affliggere l'anima di
imagini nere e spaventevoli. E questo advenne a Lucretio, philosopho epicureo, per lungo
amore; el quale prima da amore, e poi da furore di stultitia angustiato, sé medesimo
uccise'.

[37] On this subject, its sources and developments, I refer here only to the classic
Raymond Klibansky, Erwin Panofsky, Fritz Saxl, *Saturn and Melancholy. Studies in the
History of Natural Philosophy, Religion and Art* (Nendeln – Liechtenstein: Kraus Reprint,
1979).

the ethereal substrate and prompting the lover to (more or less subconsciously) reshape that mental image in a perfect form. Here, the opposite is true. The image is carved indelibly within the lover's spiritual body and cannot move beyond it and perfect it according to correct memory of the ideal. Moreover, where in the first case the lover re-shaped the specific mental image of the beloved, here the contingent image itself will reshape the physical body of the lover—and in an inferior manner, since it has been relegated to material contingency.

At this point, we might ask ourselves precisely what determines the terrible inversion of the themes seen in the preceding oration, from the wounding of the imaginative fabric to the carving of the beautiful image within the memory/heart of the lover. Ficino offers a more or less explicit answer in a passage that appears incidental, but in fact reveals that the amorous illness originates through the passage of *material* containing blood and *spiritus*, which does not take place in virtuous love. Ficino observes that

> Harmony of the other parts, with the exception of the eyes, is not the real cause of this malady, but merely provides an opportunity for it, since it invites a distant onlooker to approach, and while he is looking at close quarters, it holds him at bay before such a sight; as he watches, it is eye contact alone that inflicts the wound. But the cause of that moderate Love which participates in divinity and is the main theme of this banquet is not the eye alone: it is the harmony and comeliness of all the parts.[38]

While the beautiful proportion of the beloved's entire body gives rise to correct amorous anamnesis, an exclusive focus on the gaze results in the passage of *spiritus* and blood between beloved and lover. This is what causes bestial love. In the first case, there is no true passage of material because the sight takes in the proportion of the body; even if there is eye contact, it is not predominant and there is no opportunity for blood to be transferred. The spiritual body is not weighed down by external material

---

[38] *On the Nature of Love*, (VII-10), 149. *El libro dell'amore*, (VII-10), 205–206: 'La consonantia degli altri membri oltre agli occhi non è propria cagione, ma è occasione di tale malitia, perché tale compositione invita colui che di lunge vede che più accosto venga, e poi che di propinquo guata lo tiene a bada in tale aspecto, e mentre che bada solo el riscontro degli occhi è quello che dà ferita. Ma all'amore moderato, el quale è di divinità partefice, del quale in questo convivio comunemente si tracta, non solamente l'occhio ma etiandio la concordia e giocondità di tutte le parti come cagione concorre'.

and therefore successfully proceeds from the engraved figure of memory to locate the ideal figure hidden with the ethereal body.

Consistent with the entire seventh oration, the *remedia* proposed by Ficino involve medical and physiological cures founded on mental exercises, once again emphasising the close psychosomatic connection that characterises the human being:

> There are two methods for getting free: one is provided by nature; the other, by art. The natural method works through intervals of time, and this method is common to this malady and to all others. [...] In a similar way, the anguish of the others lasts as long as does that contagion in the blood which has been injected into the veins through the evil eye we have mentioned. [...] Once this contagion has been burned away, the unease of the foolish lovers comes to an end.[39]

As with other diseases, foreign blood is naturally consumed by the lover's body over time, freeing him from an illness that is both physical and mental. However, Ficino also proposes artificial solutions:

> To this natural method of purging must be added the work performed by very painstaking art. [...] Occasions for familiarity must be spaced out, and care must be taken above all to prevent our eyes meeting the eyes of the beloved. And if there is any defect in the soul or body of the beloved, it is to be frequently reflected upon in the mind. The soul should be given to numerous and varied matters of import; there should be regular bloodletting; wine that is clear and has a fine nose should be used; frequent bouts of intoxication will allow the old, contaminated blood to be drawn off, so that a new blood and new spirit can be produced. Regular exercise is needed, with perspiration causing the pores of the body to open and emit the unhealthy vapours, as well as regular use of foodstuffs and electuaries which physicians prescribe to cure the heart and brain. Frequent intercourse is also recommended for curing love. It received strong approval

---

[39] *On the Nature of Love*, (VII-11), 149–150. *El libro dell'amore*, (VII-11), 207–208: 'El modo dello sciorsi è di due ragioni, l'uno è della natura, l'altro è dell'arte. El naturale è quello che con certi intervalli di tempo fa sua opera, e questo modo è comune a questa malattia e a tutte l'altre [...]. Similmente l'agonia degli amanti tanto tempo dura, quanto dura quello rincerconimento del sangue, indocto nelle vene per quello male d'occhio decto. [...] Quando è chiarito tale incerconimento cessa l'affanno degli stolti amanti'.

from Lucretius when he said: "He should take pains to keep clear of decep-
tive images, throw aside the bait of love, turn his mind elsewhere, eject the
accumulated humour into various bodies, and on no account hold back the
semen once it has been contaminated by love for a particular person".[40]

Beyond the obvious suggestion of avoiding the beloved's gaze so that
further blood cannot enter, other remedies are based on artificially
removing *spiritus* and blood. Suggestions of a psychological nature—
such as thinking continuously of the defects of the beloved or dedicating
oneself to laborious tasks, so as to avoid feeding the memorial image—are
followed by physiological remedies. Ficino suggests removing old blood
and stimulating the production of new blood through the consumption
of wine. Physical exercise can also act upon the contaminated *spiritus*,
promoting its escape through the pores of the skin. It is also possible
to take action upon the heart and brain, the organs that play the most
important role in the amorous illness, through consuming specific foods
and electuaries (*'lattovari'*), that is pharmaceutical preparations. Moreover, and resorting once more to Lucretius (*De rerum natura*, IV, lines
1063–1066), Ficino states that it may be productive to have sexual rela-
tions with other people, since this will weaken the mental image of the
beloved and expel contaminated *seme*.[41]

Overall, when the strong ethical and, in places, religious tone of the
discussion of virtuous love is compared with the specifically physiological

---

[40] *On the Nature of Love*, (VII-11), 150–151. *El libro dell'amore*, (VII-11), 208–209:
'Debbesi agiugnere a questa naturale purgatione etiandio l'industria dell'arte diligentis-
sima. [...] Debbesi diradare l'usanza, e soprattutto aversi cura che gli occhi nostri non si
riscontrino, nel guatare, con gli occhi della persona amata; e se alcuno difecto è nell'animo
o nel corpo di quella, sempre nella mente rivolgerlo conviene. E appiccare l'animo a molte
diverse e gravi faccende, spesse volte trarsi el sangue e usare vino chiaro e odorifero, e
spesso innebriarsi, acciò che trahendo el sangue vecchio el quale era incerconito, si rifaccia
nuovo sangue e nuovo spirito. Usare frequente exercitatione non sudando, per le quali
e pori del corpo s'aprino a mandar fuori e vapori maligni, e frequentare ancora quegli
nutrimenti e lattovari che pongono e fisisi ad rimedio del cuore e del cervello. Ancora el
coito universale accade nella cura d'amore, al quale rimedio molto consentì Lucretio così
dicendo: «Vuolsi con diligentia fuggire le fallace imagini e levare da sé l'esca dell'amore,
e volgere la mente altrove, e gittare l'omore ragunato in diversi corpi, e in nessuno modo
ritenere el seme che per amore d'una persona è in te turbato»'.

[41] On medical practices for curing the amorous disease in the sixteenth and seventeenth
centuries, see Massimo Ciavolella, 'Eros e Memoria nella cultura del Rinascimento' in *La
cultura della memoria*, edited by Lina Bolzoni and Pietro Corsi (Bologna: Il Mulino,
1992): 319–333. For medieval practices see the classic Bruno Nardi, 'L'amore e i medici

and medical analysis of bestial love, a marked contrast is noted. Despite the importance Ficino places on the physical body of the human being and on intermediate mental faculties, the entry of physiological materiality into the amorous relationship, establishing an exchange of *spiritus* and blood between two bodies, inevitably disturbs human psychophysical balance. This disruption *overburdens* the corporeal component of the imaginative faculties and prevents anamnesis of the transcendent ideal, the true ultimate aim of the human soul. The wound of carnal love does not reveal a glimmer of the divine that lies dormant in the human being, but rather engenders psychophysical decay.

CARNALITY AS A STEPPING STONE IN *THE KISS*

Patrizi certainly inhabited a very different cultural context to that of Ficino. Where the latter addressed the so-called Accademia di Careggi, an unstructured space in which a group of co-philosophers explored the poetic *mysteries* of the *Prisca philosophia*, the former was confronted with an audience of sixteenth-century academies and the worldly northern Italian courts.[42] Patrizi is well aware that his philosophy is not destined for the wise and chaste Florentine elders, but rather a setting dominated by elegant women of high rank and courtiers well-versed in worldly questions, however much he might shun and condemn the most culturally

medievali' in Id., *Saggi e note di critica dantesca* (Milan-Naples: Ricciardi, 1966): 238–267 and Massimo Ciavolella, *La "malattia d'amore" dall'Antichità al Medioevo* (Rome: Bulzoni, 1976).

[42] On the Platonic Academy, which unlike the courts of the Cinquecento was an unstructured cultural space, see James Hankins, 'The invention of the Platonic academy in Florence,' *Rinascimento*, 41 (2001): 3–38. For the academies and kinds of courts addressed by Patrizi, see Cesare Vasoli, 'Un filosofo tra lo Studio e la Corte: Patrizi a Ferrara' in Id., *Francesco Patrizi da Cherso* (Rome: Bulzoni, 1989): 205–228, e Id., 'Le Accademie fra Cinquecento e Seicento e il loro ruolo nella storia della tradizione enciclopedica' in Id., *Immagini umanistiche* (Naples: Morano, 1983): 429–465. While Patrizi's most philosophical works are intended for the world of the universities—the *Discussiones Peripateticae* (first edition 1571) and *Nova de Universis Philosophia* (1591)—his ideological vision of establishing a new kind of intellectual figure, freed from the structures of the Counter Reformation, was aimed above all at the courts and academies; see in particular Lina Bolzoni, *L'universo dei poemi possibili. Studi su Francesco Patrizi da Cherso* (Rome: Bulzoni, 1980), 157–204; Cesare Vasoli, 'Il «Proemio» di Francesco Patrizi alla Nova de universis philosophia' in *I margini del libro. Indagine teorica e storica sui testi di dedica*, edited by Maria Antonietta Terzoli (Rome-Padua: Antenore, 2004): 77–115, 104; and Ghezzani, *Il Platonico innamorato*, especially XIX–XXXIII.

superficial and *idle* courts. Nevertheless, his broadening of Ficino's theory must not only be attributed to the changed cultural milieu, but also to the strong influence of Cinquecento *novatores*: from the intellectuals who gravitated around the Venetian Academy 'Della Fama' to the followers of Telesio.[43] Like Ficino, Patrizi initially trained as a physician, most notably at the University of Padua in the late 1540s, and his naturalistic formation is evident in many of his works, despite his supposed disappointment at the training he received in Padua.[44] Indeed, references to the teaching of two Paduan physicians, Bassiano Lando and Giovanni Battista da Monte, and his appreciation of their methodological approach seem to indicate that he preserved certain aspects of his years in the city.[45] In any case, his

---

[43] There is explicit evidence for contact between Patrizi and Tilesio—and his pupils, especially Antonio Persio—in 1572. See in particular Anna Laura Puliafito, 'La fisica telesiana attraverso gli occhi di un contemporaneo: Francesco Patrizi da Cherso' in *Bernardino Telesio e la cultura napoletana*, edited by Raffaelle Sirri and Maurizio Torrini (Naples: Guida, 1992): 257–270. On the Accademia Veneziana see the comprehensive Valeria Guarna, *L'Accademia Veneziana della Fama (1557–1561). Storia, cultura e editoria. Con l'edizione della Somma delle opere (1558) e altri documenti inediti* (Rome: Vecchiarelli, 2018).

[44] His teachers in Padua included Bernardino Tomitano, Marcantonio Passeri, Lazzaro Buonamici, and Francesco Robortello. For Patrizi's negative judgement of contemporary Aristotelianism, which is not always entirely heartfelt, see Francesco Bottin, 'Francesco Patrizi e l'aristotelismo padovano,' *Quaderni per la storia dell'Università di Padova*, 32 (1999): 163–176.

[45] In his autobiographical letter of 1587, addressed to Baccio Valori, Patrizi declares that 'towards the end of my studies I heard the physician Monte speak, and I admired his method; and the same is true of Bassiano Lando, who was his pupil at the university' (Francesco Patrizi, 'A Baccio Valori. Firenze 1587' in *Lettere ed opuscoli inediti*, 47). Monte, in particular, adopted an Aristotelian perspective but sought in his methodological works to reorganise the Hippocratic and Galenic tradition so that it could be rationally deduced, an approach that is also fundamental to Patrizi. For Monte's influence on Patrizi see Maria Muccillo, 'Dall'ordine dei libri all'ordine della realtà: ordine e metodo nella filosofia di Francesco Patrizi' in *Francesco Patrizi. Philosopher of the Renaissance*, 9–61. See also Silvia Ferretto, *Maestri per il metodo di trattar le cose. Bassiano Lando, Giovanni Battista da Monte e la scienza della medicina nel XVI secolo* (Padua: CLEUP, 2012). The earliest of Patrizi's works to be published in his first miscellaneous collection, *The Happy City* (*La città felice*), is a political discussion combined with concerns of a decidedly medical nature: see Francesco Patrizi, 'La città felice' in Id., *La città felice. Dialogo dell'honore, il Barignano. Discorso della diversità de' furori poetici. Lettura sopra il sonetto del Petrarca. La gola, e'l sonno e l'ociose piume* (Venezia: G. Griffio, 1553). On this subject see Susana Gómez López, 'Medicina y política en Francesco Patrizi: el cuerpo de La ciudad feliz,' *Asclepio. Revista de Historia de la Ciencia y de la Medicina*, 61 (2015): 1–14.

desire to re-found Ficino's thought is evident in his juvenile works and fundamentally demonstrated in the dialogue *Delfino, or the Kiss*, written at a time when he was operating in northern, and particularly Venetian, circles.

Ficino's theory, which by this date was well established among a broad, non-specialist public within the genre of love treatises, is here turned on its head—even, to a certain extent, parodied. In the wake of *On the Nature of Love*, interest in the discussion of love had developed into a widespread literary genre, represented above all by Pietro Bembo's *Asolani* (1505) and the third and fourth books of Baldassare Castiglione's *Book of the Courtier* (*Il libro del Cortegiano*, 1528). Following the philosophical focus of Leone Ebreo's *Dialogues on Love* (*Dialoghi d'amore*, 1535) and the dense Aristotelian reworking of Agostino Nifo's *On Beauty and Love* (*De pulchro et amore*, 1529)—two works which very likely influenced Patrizi—the genre stagnated through unoriginal contributions, developing into a hair-splitting subject typical of the less productive courts and academies, or discussed in didactic treatises of the Counter Reformation.[46]

Despite its tone, Patrizi's text is certainly no simple *divertissement* devoid of theoretical relevance. While the dialogue is sometimes joking and parodic, and the work concludes with a refined and graceful poetic composition, the young Patrizi's ideological mission is already well established. Employing the most typical tool of the courtly context, often used to disseminate a certain kind of philosophical knowledge, he establishes

[46] On sixteenth-century love treaties and their gradual transformation into a fashionable genre lacking any philosophical weight, see John C. Nelson, *Theory of Love: The Context of Giordano Bruno's "Eroici Furori"* (New York: Columbia University Press, 1958); Eugenio Garin, 'La filosofia dell'amore. Sincretismo platonicoaristotelico' in Id., *Storia della filosofia italiana*, vol. 2 (Turin: Einaudi, 1966): 581–615; Mario Pozzi, 'Introduzione' in *Trattati d'Amore del '500*, edited by Id. (Roma-Bari: Laterza, 1975): V–XL; Armando Maggi, 'La fase conclusiva dei trattati d'amore rinascimentali nell'autocommento poetico di Tasso' in *Indagini su Tasso. Atti del convengo internazionale. Sorrento, 6–8 novembre 2017*, edited by Alfonso Paolella (Naples: Eidos, 2018): 117–136. Also helpful for understanding the intense exchange between the love treatise genre and other Renaissance cultural phenomena is Lina Bolzoni, *Il cuore di cristallo. Ragionamenti d'amore, poesia e ritratto nel Rinascimento* (Turin: Einaudi, 2010). For an overview of the state of the field, see Delfina Giovannozzi, '«Filosofando e vagando per lo gran mare della sua essenzia». Testi e temi della trattatistica d'amore nel Rinascimento,' *Bruniana & Campanelliana*, 27 (2021): 327–333 (the introduction to a thematic section of the same title within this issue).

contact between the principal voices of the age without ever lapsing into a mere literary game of manners. Around twenty years after the composition of the *Delfino*, Patrizi, who at that time was living in Modena as a private tutor to the poet Tarquinia Molza (1542–1617), would write another dialogue on love, *The Philosophy of Love* (*L'amorosa filosofia*, 1577). In it he explicitly condemns the pedantry of 'noble courtiers and women of high rank' who deliberate the philosophy of love 'with questions and doubts and such superficial discourse – sometimes taken from Ariosto or Petrarch'.[47] Like the *Delfino*, the *Philosophy of Love* integrates complex philosophical discussion within an often witty dialogue and shares its fate as an unpublished text. The juvenile dialogue was penned during a frenetic period of Patrizi's life, characterised by multiple commitments as he sought a stable cultural base between Venice and Ferrara in the 1550s. Nevertheless, the importance of the work to its author is underlined by the fact that the only extant witness was copied by a secretary. This also implies the circulation of the text among Patrizi's acquaintances in an informal manner, with the philosopher making later corrections to both content and form.[48] Such a conclusion is also supported by the fact that Patrizi refers to the work in his *Commentary* (*Commento*) on the poetry of his friend Luca Contile.[49]

Compared to the later dialogue, the tone of the *Delfino* is markedly sharp concerning the amorous tradition, typical of the courts, that Patrizi seeks to surpass. Bembo's *Asolani* had followed in the footsteps of the *Symposium* and *Phaedrus* by gradually ascending from popular theories of love to the Platonic-Christian theory, which is revealed almost mystically by a sage hermit ('*romito*').[50] Patrizi's dialogue, however, opens differently. The young Angelo Delfino[51] has sought out Patrizi because

---

[47] Patrizi, *The Philosophy of Love*, 93 ('cortigiani gentili et gentili donne di palazzo, per via di quesiti et di dubbi o di tal discorsi superficiali et tolti dall'Ariosto o dal Petrarcha', Patrizi, *L'amorosa filosofia*, 65).

[48] For further detail see the *Critical Note*.

[49] See Patrizi, *Discorso di M. Francesco Patritio*, 17r.

[50] See Pietro Bembo, *Gli Asolani* (Florence: Accademia della Crusca, 1991), (III-11): 329–330.

[51] Establishing Delfino's identity with any accuracy is far from straightforward. In a letter to Patrizi (1562), the poet Luca Contile names Delfino among the members of the Accademia degli Affidati: 'There has been created here an Accademia degli Affidati, containing the foremost men of letters of all Italy, such as Branda, Cardano and Delfino'

he wishes to understand why the kiss is so pleasurable. The philosopher responds:

> Patr. You have given yourself poor counsel, Mr. Angelo Amoroso, that you should come to a hermit with questions about love, and one intent on other studies than those of love; for you know that the hermitage is no place for them.
>
> Del. My counsel was good, for I know that before you became a hermit you were in love; and I also know you already understand, both by proof and by learning, what love is. Therefore, prepare yourself to answer my question.[52]

Though Patrizi presents himself as a hermit, Delfino immediately brings him back down to earth, as if to remind him of the impossibility of escaping the worldly sphere. No longer the sage hermit as in Bembo's precedent, Patrizi is possessed by a knowledgeable spirit, a sort of Socratic daemon, who will speak in his place.[53] The philosopher is therefore compelled to abandon a moralising and religious tone and become a physiologist in order to provide detailed answers to Delfino's questions (through his knowledgeable spirit). Here, the kiss is presented as an aspect of love that is yet to receive a satisfactory explanation. The philosophical

---

(Luca Contile, 'A M. Franc. Patricio. 1562' in Id., *Il secondo volume delle Lettere di Luca Contile*, (G. Bartoli: Venice, 1564): 150v). However, this Delfino is not identified as the protagonist of Patrizi's dialogue, who is most likely a member of the Dolfin family, powerful players within the Venetian patriciate; see Bortolo G. Dolfin, *I Dolfin (Delfino) patrizii veneziani nella storia di Venezia dall'anno 452 al 1923* (Milan: F. Parenti, 1924). Three men named Angelo Dolfin are attested between 1535 and the early seventeenth century: Anzolo di Zuanne (1535–1595) of the Traghetto branch, Anzolo di Gerolamo (1538–1604) of the Santa Sofia branch, and Anzolo di Andrea (1545–1593) of the branch of S. Agostin Calle Bernardi.

[52] 'Patr. Non buono consiglio sarà stato il vostro, [Mr. Angelo Amoroso], di venire per amore ad huomo *romito*, et ad altri studi intento [che a gli amorosi]; [e quelli] voi sapete che nel[l']Eremo non possono haver luogo.
Del. Il mio consiglio è stato buono, per ciò che io so che avanti che voi romito diveniste foste innamorato, et so parimente che in amore, e per pr[u]ova e per iscienza, intendete avanti quanto altro qual si sia. Là onde mettetevi pure in animo di spianarmi la mia questione'.
From here on, references to the *Delfino* correspond to the edition presented in this volume and are indicated with D, followed by the relevant page number; D **50** (my italics).

[53] See D **52–53**.

tradition had discussed the question of the kiss in mystical and meta-physical terms, beginning from the kabbalistic theme of the *binsica* (or the death of the kiss) in a highly influential work that sought to present itself as a counterpoint to *On the Nature of Love*, Giovanni Pico della Mirandola's *Commentary on a canzone of Girolamo Benivieni* (*Commento sopra una canzone de amore di Girolamo Benivieni*, 1486).[54] Perhaps offering a provocative perspective on this very text, Patrizi's discussion is presented in almost exclusively earthly and physiological terms, a unicum within its genre. We might also identify a similar departure from the influential discussion of the theme of the kiss in Castiglione's *Courtier* (IV, 64), which interprets the phenomenon from an exclusively ethical perspective.[55]

In Ficino's *On the Nature of Love*, the medical-physiological tone dominates above all in the discussion of bestial love; yet here precisely the opposite is the case. Moreover, the ironic opening anticipates the complete reversal of a specifically Platonic-Christian perspective. Having established the premise that the pleasure of the kiss does not derive from the kiss itself, but rather from love for the person who is kissed,[56] Patrizi

---

[54] See Giovanni Pico della Mirandola, 'Commento sopra una canzona de amore composta da Girolamo Benivieni' in *De hominis dignitate, Heptaplus, De ente et uno, e scritti vari*, edited by Eugenio Garin (Florence: Vallecchi, 1942): 443–581, 557–558. See also the entry *Bacio* and corresponding bibliography in Giulio Busi and Raphael Ebgi (edited by), *Giovanni Pico della Mirandola. Mito, magia, qabbalah* (Turin: Einaudi, 2014), 60–72. On the philosophy of love in the exchange between Ficino and Pico, including for further bibliography, I take the liberty of referring to Tommaso Ghezzani, 'Immagini della servitù volontaria tra Marsilio Ficino e Giovanni Pico della Mirandola. Problemi di filosofia d'amore,' *Philosophia. Rivista della Società Italiana di Storia della Filosofia*, 1 (2019): 65–91.

[55] Interesting insights into the broader cultural history of the kiss are found in Nicolas J. Perella, *The Kiss Sacred and Profane: An Interpretative History of Kiss Symbolism and Related Religio-Erotic Themes* (Berkeley-Los Angeles: University of California Press, 1969), and Florence Vuilleumier Laurens, 'Les Basia de Jean Second et la tradition philosophique de Marsile Ficin à Francesco Patrizi' in *La poétique de Jean Second et son influence au xvi*^e *siècle*, edited by Jean Balsamo and Pettine Galand-Hallyn (Paris: Les Belles Lettres, 2000): 25–38. For an overview of the *Delfino* within its medical context, see above all Susana Gómez López, 'La fisiología del amor. El diálogo de Francesco Patrizi sobre los besos,' *Prometeica. Revista de Filosofía y Ciencias*, 24 (2022): 32–54; also useful is Roberta Morosini, 'Patrizi da Cherso: How and why neoplatonic kisses can give pleasure,' *Accademia. Révue de la Société Marsile Ficin*, 24 (2022): 69–84, although the proposed date is questionable (see the *Critical Note*).

[56] See D **53–54**.

sets out an exhaustive taxonomy of kisses in order of increasing pleasure, consisting of six categories (on the hands, chest, neck, cheeks, eyes,
and mouth) and four methods (with closed lips, sucking, biting, and the
tongue)[57]:

TYPE OF KISS (*increasing pleasure*)	On the hands	On the chest	On the cheeks	On the neck	On the eyes	On the mouth
METHOD OF KISS (*increasing pleasure*)	Closed lips		Biting		Sucking	With tongue

At the end of this section, it is concluded that the most pleasurable kiss
is on the mouth and with the tongue, not given but received.[58]
At this point the dialogue moves into more philosophical and physiological terrain, with a detailed analysis of the reasons for this pleasure:

D. And what is the cause of this sweetness?
P. The spirit of the beloved, which the lover consumes by kissing. [...]
I say that he who kisses invisibly consumes the spirit of the one kissed,
and this is the cause of the great sweetness that is felt in the kiss. [...]
Therefore heed what I say. We must consider two things: the first is how

---

[57] 'P. Now the amorous spirit within me commands me to tell you that amorous kisses
are given to the beloved in six places, and in four manners, and no more.
D. And what are these six places?
P. They are the hands, the chest, the neck, the cheeks, the eyes, and the mouth.
D. And the manners?
P. The manners are these: with the joining of lips, with the sucking of the lips, with
biting, and with the tongue'.
(P. Hora mi comanda lo spirito [amoroso], che è in me, che io vi dica che in sei parti
della persona amata si danno i baci [amorosi], et in quattro maniere, et non in più.
D. E quale sono queste sei parti?
P. Elle sono le mani, il petto, il collo, le guancie, gli occhi, e la bocca.
D. E le maniere?
P. Le maniere sono queste: con le labbra somme, co'l succio delle labbra, col morso,
e con la lingua (D **55**)). The differing degrees of pleasure caused by kisses upon different
parts of the body are explained at the end of the dialogue (see D **74–77**), following a
delineation of the philosophical and physiological theories that makes this possible.
[58] See D **55–58**.

love makes the spirits of the beloved pleasant, and the second is how these spirits are consumed by the lover.[59]

Here the *spiritus* resurfaces as the element that is absorbed by the lover and makes kisses pleasurable. The remainder of the dialogue will focus on explaining why the absorption of spiritual material is pleasurable and how this takes place, from a specifically physiological perspective. The solution to the first of these questions is the notion of so-called astral resemblance, or ethereal bodies, from which anamnesis of the ideal derives in an echo of Ficino's theory (analysed above). The most conspicuous difference here is that the concept of beauty is distinct from that of resemblance, while for Ficino the two are one and the same: the specific resemblance of souls is conceived as nothing other than a form of beauty. Nevertheless, some degree of concurrence between resemblance and beauty is necessary in order to bring about love, and thus the pleasure of absorbing the *spiritus* through the kiss.[60]

Proceeding to the second, weightier question—that of the physiological mechanism that makes all this possible—Patrizi draws on the motion of the *spiritus* through visual rays, comparable to that described by Ficino (Fig. 1.2) but enhanced by greater attention to particulars of the process and anatomical details:

P. The spirit, understood in a human sense, is nothing other than a most subtle vapour of the blood, which is generated in the heart by its natural heat. This spirit carries the heat of the heart through the veins, which physicians call arteries, to all of the particles of the living body, even the very smallest, which keep it hot and alive. The spirit is the true enactor of the heat and life of others; and since everything that is hot and subtle by its nature rises upwards, a large part of the spirit, which is so, rises from the body to the head and the brain, and is further purified by its

---

[59] 'D. E quale è la cagione di questa dolcezza?
P. Lo spirito dello amato, che lo amante si bee [in] baciando. [...] Io dico che chi bacia si bee [in]visibilmente dello spirito del baciato, et questa è la cagione onde nel bacio si senta cotanta dolcezza. [...] Statemi pur intento. Due cose habbiamo noi hora da vedere: l'una in qual modo amore faccia dolce gli spiriti dell'amato, e l'altra come essi si beano dallo amante' (D **58–59**).

[60] See D **59–64**. Pico had already criticised *On the Nature of Love* for describing beauty as the exterior appearance of all forms of the Good. He instead presented it as one of the many *kinds* of Good; see Pico, *Commento*, 489. See also Ghezzani, 'Immagini della *servitù volontaria* tra Marsilio Ficino e Giovanni Pico della Mirandola'.

temperature. Here, the spirit becomes an instrument not of life but of powerful knowledge of the soul and bodily movements. It is naturally sent through appropriate vessels to the instruments of sense and will, and to the nerves of motion, by which man moves and senses. Here, two vessels in the form of veins pass from the ventricles of the brain and carry the spirit that has been purified there to the eyes. Because these veins are very broad, they carry a great abundance of the spirit to the eyes; and since the spirit is itself clear, when its clarity mixes with the natural clarity of the eyes, it makes this part of animals and men bright, much more so than all the other parts.[61]

Having arrived at this point, Patrizi specifies that spiritual material does not exit through the eyes, but 'when the spirit reaches the extremities of the body, it is pushed by the beating of the heart and the movements of the limbs through little visible and hidden openings in the skin, which you men call pores, by which it exits and is dispersed. And the same occurs through openings in the eyes'.[62] In his section dedicated to *remedia amoris*, Ficino had already suggested physical exercise, without sweating, as a means to expel contaminated *spiritus* through the pores of the skin. The relevance of this detail will become clear later in the dialogue. At this juncture, it is specified how—still following Ficino's physiological model—the *spiritus* transfers blood through visual rays. With this established,

---

[61] 'P. Lo spirito, prendendolo in human significato, altro non è che un vapore sottilissimo di sangue, generato nel cuore dal natural calore di lui, il quale spirito per sue vene, che i medici addimandano arterie, porta il caldo del cuore per tutte in sino le minute particelle del vivente corpo, le quali tutte egli conserva e calde e vive. Et è vero operatore del calore e della vita altrui, et conciosia che ogni calda cosa e[t] sottile per sua natura saglia allo in su, molta parte dello spirito, che tale è, saglie dal cuore al capo et al cervello, et quivi, dalla temperatura di lui più che prima purificato, si fa stormento non della vita [più] ma delle conoscenti potenze dell'anima e de' movimenti corporali. Per ciò che egli per disposti vasi è dalla natura mandato a gli stormenti del sentire et della volontà, et a i nervi movitori, donde l'huomo si move e sente. Quivi due vasi in guisa di due vene partono da i ventricelli del cervello a gli occhi, e portano lo spirito [quivi] purgato a loro. E perché essi sono ampii assai, corre anco lo spirito per loro a gli occhi [assai] abbondante, il quale, per ciò che da se stesso è chiaro, mischiando la sua chiarezza con la naturale chiarezza degli occhi, fa negli animali e nell'huomo chiara e risplendente questa parte, più che tutte le altre parti' (D **69**).

[62] D **70**: 'lo spirito adunque, venendo alla stremità di tutto 'l corpo, e spinto dal battimento del cuore e dal movimento delle membra per quei piccioli apparenti e nascosti pertugietti della pelle, i quali voi huomini addimandate pori, se n'esce fuori e si disperde. Et il medesimo fa egli per li medesimi pertugietti degli occhi'.

P. I will demonstrate it by two proofs. The first is seen in a woman at the time of her bleeding, who upon looking into a mirror observes that it is stained with droplets of blood. This is nothing other than the spirit, which, damp with blood, is carried by the ray to the surface of the mirror, and on account of its cold temperature turns into droplets.

D. If this is true, it is a very great proof.

P. You may observe it at your leisure. I have heard several times from a philosophical spirit, who is my friend, that he demonstrated it to Aristotle, who then wrote about it in his books. But the other proof is that if one looks for any length of time into the eyes of another who is unwell, he himself will become similarly unwell.[63]

The examples of women's mirrors during menstruation (taken from Aristotle, *On Dreams* II, 459b) and the transfer of illnesses through eye contact are both taken from Ficino, who employed them in a similar argumentative context, as observed above.

In the course of the passage, the second proof is reinforced with an interesting interpretation of part of one of Petrarch's sonnets (*Canzoniere*, 233) in terms of optical physiology:

P. This, I assure you, is what happened to Petrarch when he looked into the right eye of his Laura. I know that he wrote of this in his amorous passions, and you young lovers would do well to heed it.

D. Yes, he did so in that sonnet: *Qual ventura mi fu quando dall'uno* (*What chance befell me when, from one*).

P. And this is no spell or enchantment, but rather natural force. Nature does not enact its effects without a means to do so; and between her eye and his, I know that the means was the passing of the ray and the spirit

---

[63] D 70: 'P. Da due prove manifesto il provo io, l'una delle quali è quella che si vede in donna nei tempi dei suoi sangui, la quale, mirando nel[lo] specchio, il macchia quasi di gocciole sanguigne, il che altro non è che perché lo spirito, il quale humido di quei sangui e dal raggio portato al piano dello specchio, et quivi per lo freddo di lui agghiacciando, ghioccciola diviene.

D. S'ella è vera, cotesta è grande isperienza.

P. Voi nela potete sempre a vostro diletto provare. Ma l'ho io più volte da un filosofo spirito mio amico inteso, che egli ad Aristotile il dimostrò, il quale poi ne' suoi libri lo scrisse. Ma l'altra prova si è che, s'altri mira fiso per alquanto spatio negli occhi infermi d'altrui, egli de' suoi medesimamente inferma'.

of which I speak, and that it was the spirit that carried that illness into the eye of Petrarch.[64]

The emphasis on the inextricability of literary production, philosophical knowledge, and medical knowledge, a connection already established by Ficino, anticipates the function of the elegant sonnet that will conclude the dialogue and provide a summary of its key points. In this regard, it should be recalled that the main points of *On the Nature of Love* are also summarised through the exegesis of a poetic composition, Guido Cavalcanti's (c. 1258–1300) *Donna me prega* ('A Lady asks me'), which itself had earlier been interpreted in medical terms by the physician Dino del Garbo (c. 1280–1327).[65] Pico similarly conceives his rival work of amorous philosophy as a commentary on a canzone by his friend Giro-lamo Benivieni, *Amor, dale cui man sospes'el freno* ('Love, from whose hands suspended').[66] While Fico displays an interest, typical among Tuscan authors of his time, in the tradition of the Dolce stil novo, and Pico in a particular genre of vernacular religious poetry, Patrizi demon-strates the vitality of contemporary Petrarchism, interpreting it through philosophical categories. As will later be explored in his mature decade *On Poetry* (*Della Poetica*, 1586–1588), poetry is the most fitting tool with which to unveil and communicate the deepest knowledge, as well as the best way to kindle *love* (understood in its broadest sense) within its audience. These notions are anticipated above all in the juvenile *Discourse*

---

[64] D 70–71: 'P. La qual cosa vi fo fede io essere al vostro Petrarca avvenuto dal destro occhio della sua Laura. Il che anco so che egli scrisse nelle sue amorose passioni, et voi giovani innamorati vel dovreste sapere.
D. Sì, egli è in quel sonetto: *Qual ventura mi fu quando dall'uno.*
P. E questa cosa per certo non è per incanto o per malia, ma è virtù naturale, et la natura non opera gli effetti suoi se non per alcun mezo, e, tra l'occhio di lei e quello di lui, io so che altro mezo che dagli occhi loro uscisse non fu che il raggio e lo spirito di che vi ragiono, e so che fu lo spirito quello che quella infermità recò nell'occhio del Petrarca'.

[65] See Ficino, *On the Nature of Love*, (VII-1), 132–133; *El libro dell'amore*, (VII-1), 177–179. On the interpretation of Cavalcanti by Ficino and Dino del Garbo, which move significantly beyond the text, see especially Massimo Ciavolella, 'Eros/Ereos? Marsilio Fici-no's Interpretation of Guido Cavalcanti's "Donna me prega"' in *Ficino and Renaissance Neoplatonism*, edited by Konrad Eisenbichler and Olga Zorzi Pugliese (Ottawa: Dove-house, 1986): 39–48. Dino del Garbo's commentary, in particular, represents a *summa* of treatises on erotic symptomatology from late antiquity and Arabic medicine.

[66] See Olga Zorzi Pugliese, 'Variations on Ficino's *De Amore*: The Hymns to Love by Benivieni and Castiglione' in *Ficino and Renaissance Neoplatonism*: 113–121, 113–117.

on the diversity of poetic inspirations (*Discorso della diversità de i furori poetici*, 1553), composed a few years prior to the *Delfino*.[67] Turning to a detailed exploration of how the visual rays of the beloved pass into the lover's heart, Patrizi describes the same process analysed by Ficino. While the references to Ficino's text are clear, the semantic fields of violent wounding and virulence are altogether absent, replaced instead by images relating to the harmony and friendship between spiritual substances:

> P. When the spirit exits the eye together with a luminous ray, it seeks the eye of another. […] When it blinds the other eye, it enlarges its pores, and the spirit, augmented by the force of the gaze, penetrates within. Finding that the spirits within are not enemies, but rather brothers born under the same dominium, it willingly mixes with them; and in their company, for they are just as subtle, it proceeds to seek the heart where the others were born, a place naturally dear to them and their keeper. Once the foreign spirit has been brought by the native spirit to the heart, and has subtly penetrated its substance, it inflames the heart more than ever before, and on account of the similarity it has acquired by its intimacy with the native spirits, it willingly makes its home there, as if it had returned to its proper place. This new guest is so sweet and comes from a similar and not hateful heart; so when the heart discovers it, it welcomes it and retains it gladly.[68]

---

[67] It should be noted that, a few years before the *Delfino*, Patrizi penned an erudite commentary on one of Petrarch's sonnets (*Canzoniere*, 7); see Francesco Patrizi, 'Lettura sopra il sonetto del Petrarca. *La gola, e'l sonno e l'ociose piume*', in *La città felice. Dialogo dell'honore, il Barignano. Discorso della diversità de' furori poetici. Lettura sopra il sonetto del Petrarca. La gola, e'l sonno e l'ociose piume*. On this function of poetry, which Patrizi explores and develops beginning from Ficino, see Ghezzani, *Il Platonico innamorato*, especially 137–183.

[68] D 71: 'P. Uscendo lo spirito dall'un occhio insieme col raggio luminoso, viene a ritrovare l'occhio altrui. […] Et abbagliandolo, fatti più larghi i pori suoi et aumentato lo spirito dalla forza dello affissamento, penetra dentro a loro, e ritrovando [esso] gli spiriti di là entro non nemici, ma quasi fratelli e sotto il medesimo dominio nati, si mischia con esso loro volontieri, in compagnia de' quali, sì come sottili, va diritto a ritrovare il cuore, dal quale sono quegli altri nati, sì come a luogo naturalmente caro et conservatore. Così portato lo spirito forastiero dal famigliare al cuore, e con la sottilità sua penetrando per entro la sostanza di lui, più che egli non era prima l'infiamma; et per la dimestichezza presa per la simiglianza che egli ha con li spiriti di lui famigliari, quasi in proprio luogo venuto, il si fa volontieri albergo. Et il cuore, che si truova nuovo hoste havere, sì perché egli è per sé dolce et sì perché viene da cuor simile et non odioso, ha cara la sua venuta et il ritiene volontieri'.

In contrast to Ficino, the *spiritus* of the beloved no longer wounds the heart of the lover by dangerously altering its physiological balance, contaminating its blood and constantly searching for its place of origin. Instead, a pleasant coexistence is established precisely because of the resemblance between lover and beloved (which Ficino also acknowledges), between host *spiritus* and guest *spiritus*.

The motif of specifically physiological pleasure is followed by one of mental pleasure; indeed, the two are closely connected. In *On the Nature of Love*, as we have seen, only visible recognition of the entire figure of the beloved, achieved through sight but without the exchange of *spiritus*, could trigger the memory of ideal beauty. Patrizi, on the contrary, does not hesitate to reframe Ficino's reflections on correct anamnesis within the medical-physiological context of the transfer of blood and *spiritus*:

> Moreover, since when it entered through the eyes the foreign spirit carried with it the image of beauty from which it derives, it now forms the spirits of the heart in which it dwells according to the form of beauty that it bore with it when it entered. The rational soul sees and recognises in the spirits a beauty that is very similar to the cause it has within it of the beauty of the human body, and it compares that beauty to the cause. In this comparison, it invariably happens that the contemplative soul deceives itself on account of that marvellous beauty and the loveliness of that similarity, and adds the perfection of its cause to the defects of that beauty. From this error is born a further error common to lovers, who always consider the beauty of the beloved more beautiful than it truly is.[69]

---

[69] D 71–72: 'Ma oltre, [conciosia cosa] che nell'entrata che fece lo spirito forestiero per gli occhi, con esso seco vi entra anco la imagine della bellezza donde ei deriva, egli si forma gli spiriti del cuore albergatore di quella forma che è [la] bellezza, che egli là entro portò con esso seco. La quale poi l'anima ragionevole, negli spiriti veggendo et riconoscendola in gran parte simile alla ragione che ella ha in sé della bellezza del corpo humano, la parangona con essa la ragione; nel qual paraggio sempre avviene che l'anima contemplatrice, dalla maraviglia di quella bellezza e dall'amorevolezza di quella somiglianza ingannando sé medesima, aggiunga a' deffetti della bellezza le perfettioni della ragion[e] sua. Dal qual inganno nasce poi quello inganno commune degli amanti, che più bella sempre stimano la bellezza amata, che ella non è nel vero'. This reflection on the innate ideal beauty within the soul, through which the lover unwittingly *corrects* the real appearance of the beloved, is drawn, as we have seen above, from Ficino, *On the Nature of Love*, (VI-6), 89–90; *El libro dell'amore*, (VI-6), 123.

In Ficino's macabre physiological re-reading of the *topos* of the image of the beloved within the heart of the lover, the imprinted effigy of the *spiritus* becomes an obsessive memory, the source of mania and psychophysical turbulence.[70] For Patrizi, the *spiritus* instead facilitates transcendence beyond the contingency of particular beauty, enabling the rediscovery of superior beauty. Once again, we witness a clear naturalisation of ethical and metaphysical motifs.

Nevertheless, as Ficino has already explored, external spiritual material is dispersed over time, and with it vanishes the clear image of the beloved in the memory:

> When the soul is imprinted with the beauty of another, it conserves that image safely and in its entirety for a long time. But since spirits are subtle substances, and gradually dispersed by the continued labour of the heart, when they are deprived of the sweetness of the heat of others and the sweetness of company they continuously desire to renew themselves and receive new brothers. From here is born the ardent desire to see again the eyes of the beloved[...]. But what, you will ask, causes the desire to touch the beloved? And the sweetness of the kiss?[71]

Seeing the gaze of the beloved again permits the lover to restore their *spiritus* through visual transfer, though as Patrizi has already noted such a process may also take place through the pores of the skin. This explains why physical contact generates pleasure. Coming to the crux of the entire work, he answers the question by stating:

> the heart by its nature contracts and expands, and when it expands it draws air to itself from the lungs, which in turn draw it from the nose and mouth; and it also draws in air through the whole of the skin by those small openings named pores, which lead to insensible arteries, which I termed the vessels and channels of the spirits. When the heart contracts, it

[70] See *On the Nature of Love*, (VI-9), 99–100 and (VII-8), 146; *El libro dell'amore*, (VI-9), 135–136, and (VII-8), 201–202.

[71] D **73**: 'Rimanendo l'anima stampata dalla bellezza altrui, si conserva ella per gran tempo quella imagine intera e salda. Ma gli spiriti, secondo che sono sostanze sottili et che nella continua fatica del cuore si vanno disperdendo, rimasi privi della soavità del caldo altrui et della dolcezza della compagnia, del continuo van desiderando rinovamento di sé medesimi, e nuovo ricevimento de' loro fratei carnali. Et quindi nasce l'ardentissimo desiderio di rivedere gli occhi innamora[n]ti [...]. Ma donde è, direte voi, il desiderio del toccare l'amato? E la dolcezza del baciare?'.

instead empties itself of spirits and air, and the spirits are propelled through the arteries to their mouths and arrive at the skin, where they exit the body through the said openings. The heart does this continuously while it is alive, in order to renew and refresh its spirits and its heat, which is necessary to keep it alive. [...] Since the enamoured heart is a heart, it seeks to renew its spirits; but since it is an enamoured heart, it seeks [renewal of] its joy, which is lessened and found wanting due to the dispersal of those spirits. It may be renewed by brothers of those first spirits, which may come either by seeing the eyes of the beloved again or, more abundantly, by touching the beloved person. For when the beloved is touched, the enamoured heart attempts to draw in air by natural motion by means of the arteries, but instead draws in the spirits of the beloved. Having sent them out of his heart by the same means, he draws them in instead of the air and sweetly restores himself.[72] (Fig. 1.3)

Like eye contact, physical contact permits renewal of *spiritus*, but in an even more efficient manner; and, as Patrizi states shortly afterwards, the kiss is the form of physical contact that enables its greatest reabsorption:

But now I come to the kiss. The kiss is sweet to the beloved for this reason alone: he draws to himself and consumes the spirits of the beloved, whether he kisses the hand, chest, neck, cheek, eyes or mouth. For the same reason the sucking kiss is sweeter than the joining of lips, for not only does it gather those spirits that are emitted by the beloved heart, but it draws in others by force, and all are consumed. The sucking kiss upon

---

[72] D **73–74**: 'egli per altra cagione non è che per cagione del medesimo rinovamento dello ardore e della gioia del cuore il che si fa in questa guisa: il cuore, il quale per sua natura ha movimento di ristringersi e d'allargarsi, nello allargamento che egli fa, tira l'aere in sé da' polmoni, che il tirano dal naso e dalla bocca, e tira anco l'aere da tutta la circonferenza della pelle per que' pertugetti nominati pori, a i quali finiscono insensibili arterie, ch'io dissi vasi e canali degli spiriti. Per lo contrario, nel ristringimento che il cuore fa di sé, egli si vuota degli spiriti e dell'aere tirato, et vuotandosi per lo sospingimento delle parti, corrono per le arterie gli spiriti impulsi fino alla bocca loro, finiente nella pelle, et per i pertugetti già detti s'escono del corpo. Et questo di continuo fa il cuore, mentre e' vive, per rinovamento e per rifrescamento degli spiriti suoi e del suo calore, da che è il mantenimento della sua vita. [...] Il cuore innamorato, secondo cuore, desidera rinovamento de' suoi spiriti, ma, secondo cuore innamorato, desidera rinovamento della sua gioia, la quale dal disperdimento di quei spiriti, che la gli facevano, si sciema et manca; et puotegli esser rinovata da spiriti fratelli de' primieri, e ciò li può venire o per riveduta degli occhi amati o a più copia per toccamento della persona amata. Perciò che nel toccamento di lei avviene che, tirando il cuore innamorato con moto naturale per via dell'arterie l'aria, in luogo di lei ritrovando gli spiriti dell'amato, per la medesima via mandati fuora dal cuore di lui, tira loro in vece dell'aria e soavemente se ne ristora'.

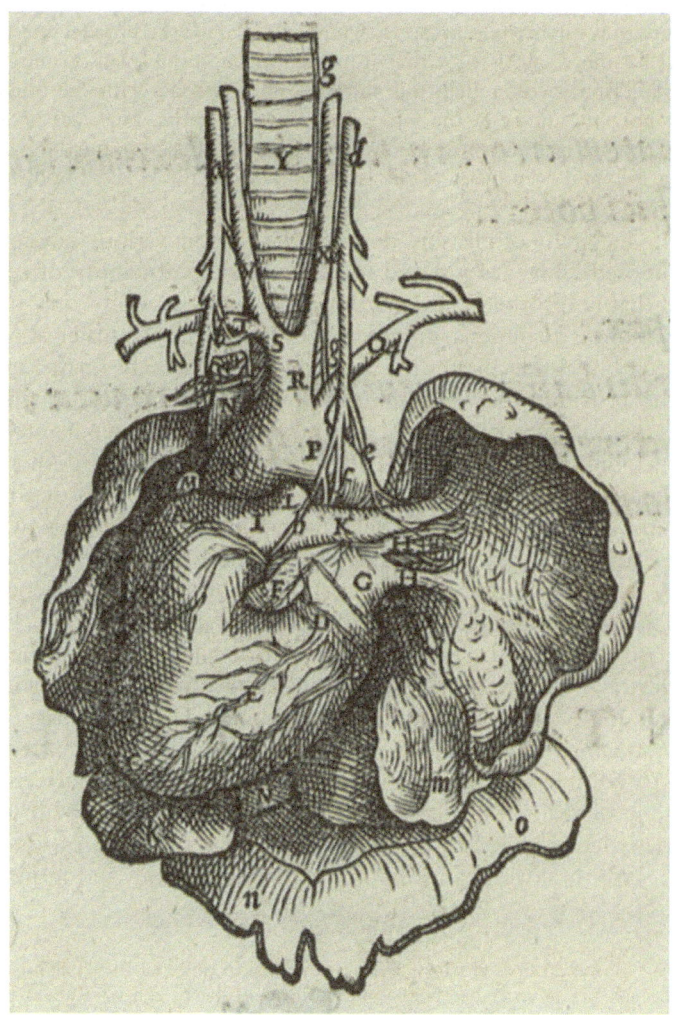

Fig. 1.3 Sixth figure of Book 6, Andreas Vesalius, *De humani corporis fabrica. Libri Septem* (Basel: J. Oporinus, 1543): 564

the mouth is furthermore sweeter than elsewhere, for the broader aperture allows for more spirits to be drawn in than through the small openings in the skin. Even sweeter than this sucking kiss is the kiss with the tongue, for it not only draws in the same abundance of spirits, but a far greater number, since it draws in those of the tongue, which is a spongy body and always full, and even tastes of the inner humour of the beloved body.[73]

Here, the hierarchy of pleasure derived through the various categories of kiss, proposed above, is justified in relation to the quantity of spiritual material that is absorbed. This physiological permeation not only permits correct amorous anamnesis, unimpeded by the material transfer of organic substances, but also facilitates the rebalancing of the body, further emphasising the proximity between the physical and psychic-rational spheres. Indeed, the anamnestic act would seem to require greater mental force than acts of an ordinary nature. The *spiritus* of the beloved both enables and maintains anamnesis, not corrupting the other powers of the soul but on the contrary allowing them to support this operation without causing damage. In Ficino, however, the permeation of *spiritus* corrupts not only fantasy and memory, but also physiological balance, generating the melancholic humours of the love illness.

The conclusion to the text offers further details concerning the other categories of the kiss, among which the 'kiss with biting' is particularly significant for our investigation. Patrizi reprises Ficino's theory of the *vendetta amorosa* but does away with the pathological violence that characterised it. While for Ficino the mad bestial lover is characterised by excessive passion for the beloved, sometimes accompanied by an unconscious destructive violence, Patrizi explains that this type of kiss takes place because the lover, 'since he burns for that person, and in his heart

---

[73] D 75: 'Ma vengo hora al bacio. Egli non è per altro dolce [il bacio] all'innamorato che perché egli tira in sé et bee degli spiriti dell'amato, bacisi egli o mano, o petto, o collo, o guancia, od occhi, o bocca. Per la qual stessa cagione il bacio del succio è più dolce che non è quello delle supreme labbra, perciò che non solo egli si raccoglie quelli che sono del cuore amato mandati fuora, ma con la forza del tiro se ne tira egli degli altri a forza, e tutti se gli bee. D'onde anco è che più degli altri succi è dolce il succio della bocca, perché per quindi, come per più larga via, molti più ne tira, che per quei piccioli pertugietti della pelle. D[i] questo bacio del succio è anco più dolce il bacio della lingua, conciosia cosa che egli non solo tira quella medesima copia degli spiriti che 'l succio, ma la si tira egli molto maggiore di lui, perciò che egli si tiri quelli della lingua ancora, la quale è tutta spongioso corpo et n'è del continuo ripiena, et anco gusta dell'interior humore del corpo amato'.

is offended by her, he is compelled by a sudden desire for revenge on she who possesses him, and he takes up those arms that are most ready. But realising that he has life through her, he swiftly repents and turns that revenge to sweet nourishing of his flames'.[74] There is a hint of affront about the lover, who in a certain sense has lost the individual liberty he possessed before falling in love; but this situation is easily overcome through his progress towards knowledge of the greater good, transforming the desire for revenge into an erotic game.

The dialogue closes with the voice of Delfino, who, enlightened by new and deep knowledge, is no longer ignorant but wise. Having reached the cognitive climax, and almost as if he in turn has been possessed by an amorous spirit, he *gives birth* to a sonnet summarising the key points of the dialogue. Pregnant with knowledge, he echoes Diotima, for whom the lover is revealed 'to give birth in beauty'[75] on the part of the beloved. Delfino conclusively demonstrates, as has been anticipated, that poetry plays a privileged role in allowing us to approach and articulate true love of knowledge, in which the body also necessarily participates.[76]

In conclusion, even in this early text it is clear that Patrizi adopts a position utterly at odds with Ficino's paradigm of love. In Ficino's model, the entry of external blood wounded the heart, resulting in contamination of the blood and *spiritus* and, consequently, the fantasy and memory, establishing a vicious circle. Only removal of that blood by natural or artificial means could restore the complex psychosomatic balance. For Ficino, correct amorous anamnesis—despite the fact that it was always initiated by action on the spiritual-imaginative fabric—could only take place through visual experience without any form of material transfer between lover and beloved. Patrizi reformulates this model, broadening the sphere of legitimate physical experience and thus transforming the contiguity and collaboration between soul and body: an aspect on which

---

[74] D 76: 'raccordatosi che egli arde per quella persona, et è da lei nel cuore offeso, spinto da un subbito desiderio di vendetta in quella che [la] possiede, adopra quelle armi che più preste gli sono. Ma ricordatosi che egli ha anco vita per lei, prestamente pentito volge quella vendetta in dolce nutrimento delle sue fiamme'.

[75] Plato, *Symposium*, edited by A. Sharon (Newburyport: Focus Publishing, 1998), (206b), 56.

[76] For further consideration of the implications of this poetic conclusion, I take the liberty of referring to Ghezzani, *Il Platonico innamorato*, 74–77.

Ficino had insisted, albeit without deriving such strong naturalistic repercussions.[77] Here, carnal love—consisting not only of the exchange of spiritual material between lover and beloved through the gaze but also, and above all, through touch—is recognised as a cure for the body, for physical memory and for metaphysical anamnesis. The spiritual arrow wounds the heart of the lover, carving its image upon the imaginative canvas, but this does not impede the rediscovery of latent ideal beauty; rather, it makes such a process possible and, at the same time, maintains the balance of the body. For Ficino, the sight of particular earthly beauty was capable of directing thought towards universal perspectives, on account of the analogic mirroring of all degrees of the real that is implicit in his metaphysics. In the same way, Patrizi shows how in the context of love the material should not be excluded from the positive trajectory of the analogic chain of being. Even carnality, if correctly employed, may help realise the ultimate goal of the human soul,[78] and thus a medical-physiological text may become a stepping stone towards ethical and metaphysical aims.

These elements represent the distinctive traits of Patrizi's entire philosophy of love, which would later be further developed in his *Discourse* on Contile's poetry and the mature dialogue *The Philosophy of Love*.[79] In this

---

[77] Nevertheless, Patrizi remains broadly within the bounds of Platonism, in both this text and his entire production. The Aristotelian tradition also witnesses reworkings of the philosophy of love as derived from Plato along naturalistic lines; see for instance the aforementioned Agostino Nifo, *De pulchro et amore* (Rome: A. Blado, 1529).

[78] In the *Delfino*, too, the potential abuse of carnal love is briefly discussed at D **64**.

[79] For a contextualisation of the *Discorso*, see Luciana Borsetto, '«Concetti da porre in amorosa poesia». L'*accessus* neoplatonico del Patrizi alle Rime di Luca Contile' in Ead., *Riscrivere gli Antichi, riscrivere i Moderni e altri studi di letteratura italiana e comparata tra Quattro e Ottocento* (Alessandria: Edizioni dell'Orso, 2002): 303–320. For a study centred more on the rhetorical and linguistic theme of the work, see Ester Pietrobon, 'Gli *Argomenti* di Francesco Patrizi come teatro ermeneutico del testo' in *Canzonieri in transito. Lasciti petrarcheschi e nuovi archetipi letterari tra Cinque e Seicento*, edited by Alessandro Metlica and Franco Tomasi (Milan-Udine: Mimesis, 2015): 37–58. It is important to consider the historiographical debate around the *Amorosa filosofia*. The work's first editor considered the theory of *philautia*, the focus of the work, to be the primary point of distinction from the model of Ficino (see James C. Nelson, '«L'amorosa filosofia» di Francesco Patrizi da Cherso,' *Rinascimento*, 2 (1962): 89–106), a position shared by Cesare Vasoli, '«L'amorosa filosofia»: dall'«amore platonico» all'universale «philautia»' in *Francesco Patrizi da Cherso*: 181–204, and Muccillo, *Marsilio Ficino e Francesco Patrizi*, 640–647. However, this opinion requires reconsideration, as observed Igor Škamperle, 'L'*amorosa filosofia* di Frane Petrić e il concetto di *Philautia*,' *Prilozi*, 75 (2012): 23–34,

regard, there is clearly continued relevance in the long-standing claim that 'when we come to look more closely at the ethics of love at the time of the Renaissance, we are struck by a remarkable contrast'. It is a contrast between the immoderate hedonism of the storytellers and comic poets and the spirituality of the lyric poets and authors of dialogues, and yet, 'it is a fact, that, in the cultivated man of modern times, this sentiment can be not merely unconsciously present in both its highest and lowest stages, but may thus manifest itself openly, and even artistically. The modern man, like the man of antiquity, is in this respect too a microcosm'.[80]

CRITICAL NOTE

The text is based on the sole extant witness, Milan, Biblioteca Ambrosiana ms. Q 119 sup. (fols. 106r–117v), from the collection of G. V. Pinelli. The codex is a miscellany of short works by various authors, including several of a natural philosophical and alchemical nature; the presence of Patrizi's work on love is straightforwardly explained by its attention to the notions of the *spiritus* and ethereal body. The manuscript is undated and its antegraph has not survived. It is copied in the hand of a secretary, with numerous corrections in Patrizi's own hand, often substantial. In addition to orthographic and morphological amendments, he erases large sections, rewriting them and adding large tracts of new material. For the most part, such alterations are of a stylistic nature (Fig. 1.4).

The manuscript is in reasonable condition, with only two exceptions: tears to the lower part of folio 106, which has been repaired on both sides with adhesive tape, and the lower corner of folio 113.

and Erna Banić-Pajnić, 'Marsilio Ficino and Franciscus Patricius on Love' in *Francesco Patrizi. Philosopher of the Renaissance*: 213–231. On the whole, and despite the claims of the characters of the dialogue, *philautia* is much more an aspect of Ficino's thought than has been admitted; see for instance Ficino, *El libro dell'amore*, (VI-19), 175. The key distinctions are more likely to be found in the first section of the work—often and unfairly overlooked in the historiography—where the strongly naturalistic angle of Patrizi's analysis continues to emerge. Useful in this regard are Maria Giovanna Cavallari, 'L'insegnamento del Patrizi in alcuni madrigali di Tarquinia Molza' in *Francesco Patrizi. Filosofo platonico nel crepuscolo del Rinascimento*: 129–138, Sandra Plastina, 'Is Francesco Patrizi's *L'Amorosa Filosofia* a heterodox reading of the *Symposium*?,' *Intellectual History Review*, 29 (2019): 631–648, and Ghezzani, *Il Platonico innamorato*, 123–137, all of which focus precisely on the opening section.

[80] Jacob Burckhardt, *The Civilization of the Renaissance in Italy* (Vienna: Phaidon Press, 1954), 229.

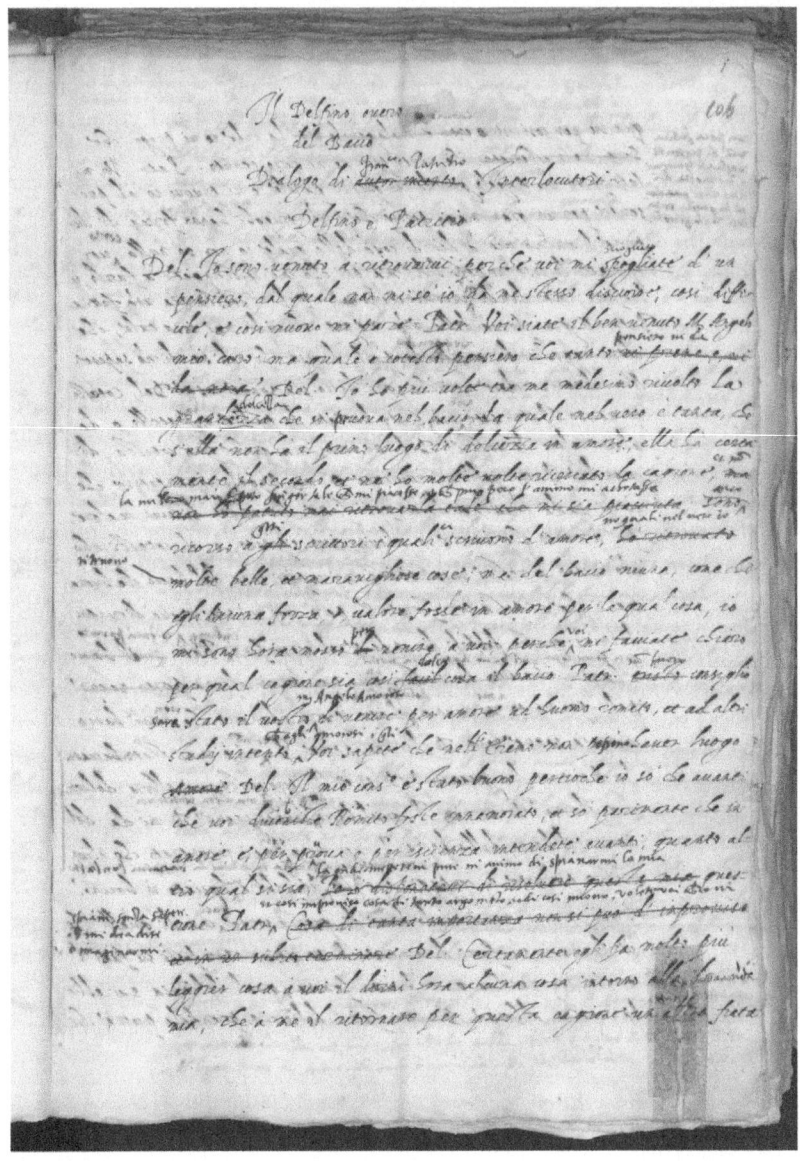

Fig. 1.4 First folio of the manuscript: MS Q 119 sup., fol. 106r, Milan, Biblioteca Ambrosiana

These do not compromise the reading. Patrizi's interventions are made in slightly lighter ink than that used by the secretary. For a more detailed description of the codex see Paul O. Kristeller, *Iter Italicum*, vol. 1 (London – Leiden: Brill, 1963): 308–309, and Adolfo Rivolta, *Catalogo dei codici pinelliani dell'Ambrosiana* (Tipografia Pontificia Arcivescovile S. Giuseppe: Milan, 1933): 58–60.

The edition has been prepared with every effort to maintain the author's final will. The critical apparatus—which is positive, since it concerns a *codex unicus*—details the version of the text prior to Patrizi's corrections and additions, with the original secretarial text that was modified or expunged in regular characters. Editorial comments are given in round brackets, where relevant. Within the text itself, Patrizi's amendments are denoted with square brackets; in the manuscript, they are generally indicated with an inverted *v* or written directly above the secretarial text. Also within the text, round brackets are used for folio numbers (in bold type) and braces introduce the few editorial additions, which are generally minor and of a grammatical nature.

The transcription follows a principle of minimal intervention. Adjustments are limited to modernisation of punctuation, capitalisation, and expansion of abbreviations. The original spelling has otherwise been maintained: it essentially follows a humanistic mimicry of Latin etymologies (initial *h*, *ti* for *zi*, etc.), with corresponding fluctuations.

The present work seeks to present a more trustworthy critical edition than the only previous published version of the text, edited by Danilo Aguzzi Barbagli in the collection *Lettere ed opuscoli inediti* (Florence 1975, 135–164). Among the numerous defects of this edition, some significant, we note:

1. Inconsistent alternation between excessive orthographic and morphological modernisation and the preservation of original forms, despite the editor's claims to make minimal alterations to the original spelling (*Lettere ed opuscoli inediti*, XXXII).
2. Shortcomings in the critical apparatus. The editor claims he will follow the earlier version of the text predating Patrizi's corrections (*Lettere ed opuscoli inediti*, 135), but in reality the approach is inconsistent and transcription errors are not infrequent.
3. Confusion between certain words and the unjustified omission of individual words and entire expressions. These editorial errors are particularly serious because in places they alter the sense of Patrizi's

discourse. Among the most egregious errors we note: the omission of two entire lines (here p. 54); *nari* for *mani* (p. 55); *bontà* for *bevuta* (p. 58); *insensibilmente* for *invisibilmente* (p. 67); the omission of two crucial lines, the absence of which completely distorts the proposed definitions of *desiderio, affettione,* and above all *amore* (p. 63); and *nostro* for *vostro* along with derived forms (various occurrences).

4. The problem of the work's date. In the introduction to *Lettere ed opuscoli inediti,* the editor attributes the dialogue to Patrizi's mature period, more specifically 1577 during his sojourn in Modena, thus making it contemporaneous with *L'amorosa philosophia*: 'This supposition is based on the fact that, in the *Delfino,* Patrizi assumes an intellectual position so close to that underpinning *L'amorosa filosofia* that we are compelled to consider the first dialogue an inevitable completion of the second' (*Lettere ed opuscoli inedita,* XXIII). This judgement is based on little textual insight and fails to take into account Patrizi's reference to his work on the kiss in his *Commento* on the *Rime* of Luca Contile (written in 1560) (*Commento,* fol. 17r: 'similarly, none other than the lover may judge the pleasure of this savouring. This is shown in the kiss, and in its many forms, as I have set out on a previous occasion'). On a formal level, moreover, the systematic nature and stylistic elegance of the *Delfino* are typical of Patrizi's earlier period, beginning with his first collection of short works published in Venice in 1553. This formal hallmark is lacking in his later production, with the sole exception of the mature *Philosophy of Love.* In terms of content, it must also be noted that the entire theory, presented in the *Delfino,* of the descent of the soul through the celestial spheres bears strong similarities with a similar discussion in the *Discourse on the diversity of poetic inspiration,* a short text included in the Venetian collection of 1553. Curiously, these aspects were not unknown to Aguzzi Barbagli, who on their basis attributed the *Delfino* to a more realistic period between 1553 and 1560 in a contribution published a few years before his edition of the text ('Un contributo di Francesco Patrizi da Cherso alle dottrine rinascimentali sull'amore,' *Yearbook of Italian Studies,* 2 (1972): 19–50). Other than the superficial consideration mentioned above, it is unclear what led the editor to so radically alter his opinion regarding the dating of the *Delfino,* abandoning his solid reasoning of a few years earlier.

Lina Bolzoni has commented on the issues in Aguzzi Barbagli's work in a detailed review, where she provides a clear table of the editor's many transcription errors ('A proposito di una recente edizione di inediti patriziani,' *Rinascimento*, 16 (1976): 133–156). In preparing this edition, we have drawn on her observations, above all in relation to the period of the work's composition, to which we refer for further detail concerning its possible date ('A proposito di una recente edizione,' 148–149).

One further edition of the *Delfino* is based on that of Aguzzi Barbagli, namely the French translation of Sylvie Laurens Aubry (*Du baiser*, Paris 2002). This edition, whose editor is clearly unaware of Bolzoni's review, inherits many of Aguzzi Barbagli's errors: only nine (ibid., 90) are corrected of a much larger number.

Translator's Note

I have endeavoured to balance fidelity to the semantic precision of Patrizi's terminology with the conversational and often witty tone of the dialogue. Where possible, I have avoided dramatic alterations to syntax so as to facilitate comparison of the translation and original text. I trust that readers will consider such an approach to be consistent with the motivations behind this critical edition, and indeed behind Patrizi's own composition of the *Delfino*.

Matthew Coneys

CHAPTER 2

(106r) Il Delfino, overo del Bacio

DIALOGO DI FRANCESCO PATRITIO.[1] INTERLOCUTORI:
DELFINO E PATRITIO

DEL. Io sono venuto a ritrovarvi, perché voi mi sciogliate[2] d'un pensiero, dal quale non mi so io da me stesso disciorre, così difficile e così nuovo mi pare.

PATR. Voi siate il ben venuto, Mr. Angelo mio caro; ma quale è cotesto pensiero, che tanto pensiero vi dà?[3]

DEL. Io ho più volte tra me medesimo rivolto la gran[4] [dolcezza] che si pruova[5] nel bacio, la quale nel vero è tanta, che s'ella non ha il primo luogo di dolcezza in amore, ella ha certamente il secondo, et ne ho molte volte ricercato la cagione, et non la mi sono mai saputo finger tale che mi piacesse, et per poco l'animo mi achetasse.[6] Sono [anco] ricorso a quelli[7]

---

[1] *di* autore incerto

[2] spogliate

[3] *che tanto* vi preme, e, vi dà noia

[4] *grand*ezza

[5] tr*uova*

[6] *la cagione*, ma non ho potuto mai ritrovarla tale che mi sia piaciuta

[7] *a* gli

T. Ghezzani, *The 'Kiss' and the Medicine of Love*, Palgrave Studies in Medieval and Early Modern Medicine, https://doi.org/10.1007/978-3-031-75283-4_2

49

scrittori, i quali [ci] scrivono d'amore, ne' quali nel vero io ritrovo[8] molte belle et maravigliose cose; ma del bacio niuna, come che egli di niuna forza, o valore, fosse in amore. Per la qual cosa io mi sono hora mosso per[9] venire a voi, perché [voi] mi facciate chiaro per qual cagione sia così dolce[10] cosa il bacio.

PATR. Non buono[11] consiglio sarà stato il vostro, [Mr. Angelo Amoroso], di venire per amore ad huomo romito, et ad altri studi intento [che a gli amorosi]; [e quelli] voi sapete che nel[l']Eremo non possono haver luogo.[12]

DEL. Il mio consiglio è stato buono, per ciò che io so che avanti che voi romito diveniste[13] foste innamorato, et so parimente che in amore, e per pr[u]ova e per iscienza, intendete avanti quanto altro qual si sia. Là onde mettetevi pure in animo di spianarmi la mia questione.[14]

PATR. Et così improvviso cosa di tanto argomento, e di così nuovo, volete voi che vi spiani, senza sapere che mi dea dire o imaginarmi.[15]

DEL. Certamente egli fia molto più leggier cosa a voi il dirmi hora alcuna cosa intorno alla domanda mia, che a me il ritornare per questa cagione un'altra fiata (**106v**) qua su per così aspro camino,[16] là onde io vi prego, che con poca fatica vostra, di presente vogliate levarne a me molta di ritornare in su questa erta così malagevole,[17] che tanto più ve ne sarò tenuto.

PATR. Voi mi fate forza, Mr. Angelo gentile, con queste parole, e vi pruovo io al presente per un gran mago poscia che i vostri prieghi hanno forza di disporre l'animo mio a dir di cosa della quale io non so nulla.

---

[8] *d'amore,* ho ritrovato

[9] di

[10] facil

[11] Tristo *consiglio*

[12] *non* può *haver luogo* Amore

[13] *che voi* diveniste romito (the inversion is indicated by the insertion of ·b· and ·a· above *diveniste* and *romito* respectively)

[14] Però disponetevi di risolvere questa mia *questione*

[15] Cosa di tanta importanza non si può d'improviso e in un subito esaminare

[16] *aspra* erta, e, malagevole via

[17] *vi prego, che* hora me n'esponiate, *che tanto più* (within the amendment, the word *quasi* has been deleted between *ritornare* and *in su*)

[Certo] voi operate le cose impossibili, ma poi che mi constringete a farlo, io lo farò. Ma donde [io m'] incomincierò?[18]

DEL. Cotesta sia vostra fattica.

PATR. O gran forza della vostra magia. Chi mai udì cosa tale, che altri vegghiando et veggendo[19] parli di cosa che egli sa di non sapere. Ma ditemi, credete voi che ogni bacio sia soave cosa?

DEL. Cotesto io non so.

PATR. Sete [voi] mai stato baciato da padre, o [da] fratello, o da alcun altro de' vostri?

DEL. Sì sono. Ma a che fine cotesta dimanda?

PATR. Egli mi conviene, o Mr. Angelo incantatore, che io vi vada trattenendo con così fatte dimande di niun valore, fin a tanto che Amore, o alcuno suo spirito, o di cotesti che obediscono a' vostri incantesimi, mi ispiri cosa del bacio che buona sia e che vi possa sodisfare, e però non vi sia grave di rispondermi a queste debboli dimande.

DEL. Così farò io adunque.

PATR. Et evvi paruto così soave cosa quel bacio datovi da' vostri?[20]

DEL. Per certo a me niuna[21] dolcezza ha dato.

PATR. Pare adunque che [non] ogni bacio sia[22] soave cosa.

DEL. Così pare.

P. [Et non] vi è mai stata baciata la fronte o la guancia?

D. Sì è.

P. [Et] provaste voi alhora dolcezza alcuna?

D. Io no.

P. Bacio adunque di qual maniera sentite voi soave?[23]

D. Mi dà dolcezza il bacio della bocca.

---

[18] *incomincierò* io?

[19] vedendo

[20] Quel bacio ch'avete ricevuto da' vostri evvi paruto in alcuna parte soave? (Patrizi adds a *v* to *evvi*)

[21] *Per certo* in *niuna*

[22] non *sia*

[23] Qual *bacio* sentite *soave*?

P. Non vi è [egli] mai incontrato che alcun parente vostro,[24] o compagno, o amico, [sì come havete voi a Vinegia in costume di baciarvi l'un l'altri per la via], vi habbia [mai] baciato in bocca?

D. Sì. Ma io non intendo di questa sorte baci[25] ma di quelli che si danno in su fatti d'amore.

P. Se voi a caso foste su fatti d'amore con vecchia, o con brutta femina, [o con alcuna a cui putisse il fiato], qual dolcezza sarebbe la vostra alhora?

D. Così fatta dolcezza prendala pure chi (**107r**) vuole, che per me non ne beo.

P. Ma sì bevete voi di baci di bella donna?[26]

D. Di cotesti sì bene.[27]

P. Pure credete voi ch'ogni bacio d'ogni bella donna sia soave cosa?

D. Crederò [io][28] che sì.

P. Io ho sentito più volte a molti giovani [generosi] dire che, quando essi sono in su fatti amorosi[29] con commune femina, quantunque bella, essi fuggono in tutto il bacio; quasi vi sentissero entro schifezza anzi che dolcezza.

D. Cotesto io non so s'io mi dea credere così de leggieri; ma in[30] bacio di persona amata che direte voi che avenga?

P. O gran providenza di Amore, come ci hai tu da cose vane[31] condotto alle tue meraviglie?[32] Veramente che di te[33] questa solitudine è piena, e[t] pieno è questo aere de' tuoi santi spiriti. Eccovi, Mr. Angelo amoroso, che io mi riempio di spiriti amorosi, i quali mi dett[er]a[n]no dolci dettati da risolvere la vostra dolce et amorosa questione. E però tu, o molto

---

[24] vostro parente (the inversion is indicated by the insertion of ·b· amd ·a· above *vostro* and *parente* respectively)

[25] baci *di questa sorte* (above the deleted *baci* is another, illegible deletion)

[26] Se voi beveste di quella de' baci *di bella donna?* (above the deleted *beveste* is another, illegible deletion. The first *di* of the sentence is added by Patrizi)

[27] Di questa me ne pascerei io bene e volontieri. (*io* probably corrects a barely legible *sì*)

[28] (*io* is repeated twice, probably because the first addition, which is very small and almost at the edge of the page, seemed insufficient to Patrizi)

[29] d'*amore*

[30] nel

[31] *vane* e di niun valore

[32] altissime *meraviglie*

[33] (the word substituted by *di te* is unclear)

da me riverito e venerato Amore, desta in me i tuoi spiriti, et questo hoggimai nella solitudine raffreddato mio cuore raccendi, perché io possa convenevole alle tue divine fiamme questo amoroso giovane delle tue maravigliose, et ineffabili forze raguagliare. Et così pregatel anco voi, Mr. Angelo mio, che egli a noi sia in questa giornata et sempre propitio e favorevole.

D. Et così io nel prego, ma voi rispondente alla mia dimanda.

P. Io credo che dolcezza ineffabile si pruovi in[34] bacio di persona amata. Et hora mi detta lo spirito, che m'empie il cuore,[35] che nulla altra cosa è che faccia soavità nel bacio che amore, senza il[36] quale il bacio è morta et insoave cosa.[37]

D. Et in qual guisa è cotesto?

P. Io [i]l [vi] dirò,[38] ma voi non contrastate allo spirito, che hora parla in me, per ciò ché egli è buono spirito, et non è per mentirvi.

D. [Io] così farò, [ma voi seguite pure].

P. Il bacio delle difformi donne è schifo, non è così?

D. Così è certamente.

P. Quello de' parenti e degli amici né schifo, né ha quella dolcezza di che noi parliamo, la quale è nell'amoroso solo.[39]

D. È vero.

P. Sì come[40] niuna cosa arde o riscalda, se non per il fuoco, così niun bacio è condito di dolcezza, se non l'amoroso. Non è così?[41]

D. Sì è il vero.[42]

---

[34] nel

[35] *il cuore* d'affetto,

[36] de*l*

[37] *il quale* né soavità, né altro ben si pruova.

[38] Ve *lo dirò*

[39] *degli amici,* non è *né schifo, né* dolce, ma come cosa vuota d'effetto. (the first *e* of *effetto* corrects an *a*)

[40] Possiam dunque dire che *sì come* (the mark Patrizi uses to integrate additions is present at the beginning of the line, but there is no interpolation)

[41] *per il fuoco* che ha in se stessa, che *così niun bacio* può esser dolce, *se non* è condito d'amore. (*d'amore* corrects *con l'amore*)

[42] Gli è *il vero,* per ciò che se'l (**107v**) bacio per sua natura fosse dolce, e portasse seco la soavità che si sente, seguirebbe che in ciascuna persona ei sarebbe soave et dolce, cosa che non può essere (*può essere* is corrected with another phrase that has in turn been

[P. Amore adunque è quello che mette dolcezza nel bacio, per questo senza amore è privo di dolcezza, sì come il legno privo di fuoco non arde o riscalda.

D. Voi dite il vero.]

(107v) Pa. Non è adunque il bacio per sua natura quello che dia dolcezza, poiché se egli con esso seco portasse da natura sua la soavità, da qual si voglia persona che si porgesse egli sempre soave sarebbe, il che però non avviene, poiché esso è anco schiffo, et altro è né questo né quello.[43]

D. Così sta nel vero.

P. Non altra cosa è adunque che amore la quale ponga nel bacio la dolcezza, poscia che solo quel bacio è soave[44] che è tra persone amanti, [siccome solo quel legno riscalda che ha in sé di fuoco.]

D. Per certo ci detta vero cotesto spirito che vi è entrato in cuore.

P. Il bacio adunque condito nelle dolcezze d'amore porge a gli[45] amanti quella soavità ineffabile, che essi [in] baciando l'un l'altro si prova[no.]

D. Solo questo il fa.

P. Ma è egli[46] possibile, Mr. Angelo mio, che voi non proviate dolcezza in altro bacio amoroso veruno che[47] in quello della bocca?

D. In quello della guancia ancor io la sento, ma non sempre di lunga possa.[48]

P. Et in bacio d'altra parte?[49]

D. [Et di] qual altra?[50] Poiché quello della fronte non è bacio amoroso ma di pura amorevolezza del maggiore.

---

deleted and is hardly legible); però credo che non il bacio ma amore sia quello che causa questa dolcezza.

[43] P. Chiara cosa è che il bacio per sua natura non è quello che dia dolcezza, per ciò che, se egli con esso seco portasse la soavità a qual si voglia persona che ei (ei is corrected but the subsituted term is unclear) si porgesse, egli sempre soave sarebbe, il che però non avviene, perché alcuno è schifo, alcuno né schifo né dolce.

[44] la dolcezza, per ciò che si vede che solo quel bacio è soave

[45] alli

[46] È possibile

[47] amoroso salvo che

[48] Io la provo ancora in quello della guancia ma non così grande. (above io la provo is another illegible deleted correction)

[49] P. Nel baciar altra parte?

[50] Qual altra parte?

P. Pregate, pregate Amore che egli vi mostri e scuopra tutti i segreti della sua dolcezza, per ciò che senza la gratia sua voi non ardirete neanco[51] di mirare nel profondo abisso delle sue dolcezze.

D. [Et] io così di tutto cuore [divotamente] il pr[i]ego, che egli mi faccia degno consideratore di suoi maravigliosi et ineffabili piaceri.

P. Hora mi comanda lo spirito [amoroso], che è in me, che io vi dica che in sei parti[52] della persona amata si danno i baci [amorosi], et in quattro maniere, et non in più.

D. E quale sono queste sei parti?

P. Elle sono le mani, il petto, il collo, le guancie, gli occhi, e la bocca.

D. E le maniere?

P. Le maniere[53] sono queste: con le labbra somme, co'l succio delle labbra, col morso, e con la lingua.

D. Io ti ringratio, o Amore, che me ne fai capace, et così ti riprego per la tua benignità che tu mi prosperi ne' tuoi segreti. Ma tu, o spirito che sei nel cuore del Patritio, degnati a dichiararmi (**108r**) queste cose ad una ad una.

P. Così farò. Delle parti, [o Mr. Angelo], la meno dolce a baciare sono le mani, più di loro è dolce il petto. [Et è gran cosa a dire quella che io vi voglio dir hora], che essendo il petto parte più molle e più delicata che non è il collo, [nondimeno più soavità si prova in baciando il collo, che in baciando il petto non si fa], et è tanta la dolcezza in questo bacio del collo, che se ella non agguaglia quelle delle guancie, che pur sono in gran parte albergo della bellezza, per certo di poco spazio ella le va dietro.[54]

D. Voi dite vero[55] ch'ella è grande la dolcezza che è nel bacio del collo, ma ch'egli così stia in paragon delle gote io il crederò a te, o spirito amoroso, per ciò che pruova non ne ho fatto.[56]

---

[51] *manco*

[52] *parte*

[53] *Le maniere* del baciar

[54] *è dolce il petto*, più del petto è dolce il collo, *che essendo il petto* molto *parte più molle e più delicata che non è il collo*, ci porge minor soavità del baciare. *È tanta la dolcezza* di *questo bacio del collo, che se ella non agguaglia quelle delle guancie, che pur sono in gran parte albergo della bellezza, per certo di poco spazio ella* se ne resta a*dietro.*

[55] (This sentence, added in its entirety by Patrizi above the deletion, contains a deleted *il* between *dite* and *vero*)

[56] Questa cosa mi pare impossibile, ma non ne havendo fatto pruova la credarò a te, *o spirito*, che con tanto amore ragioni.

P. Se voi ne la farete, sentirete[57] essere vero quello che io vi dico. Il bacio degli occhi è dolcissimo, ma il bacio della bocca [è quel bacio] {che} supera[58] et avanza la dolcezza di tutti gli altri baci, ancora che posti insieme.[59]

D. Di questo, o spirito buono, io non n'ho dubbio.

P. Et sapete[60] questo bacio della bocca è[61] di quattro maniere, l'una più dell'altra soave et dolce.[62]

D. E quali sono elle?

P. Per congiongimento de' labbri a' labbri, per succio de' labbri amati, col porgere la lingua e col riceverla.

D. Tu di'[63] vero, e questa io stimo la maggior dolcezza che [in bacio] si possa sentire.[64]

P. Ma voi non ponete mente, o Delfino, ad una gran differenza[65] che è tra questo bacio della bocca a gli altri baci.

D. Io no[66] per certo, ma quale è ella?

P. Tutti gli altri baci, o siano in mano, o in petto, o in collo, o in gote, o in occhi si danno; ma quello della bocca [solo et] si dà e si riceve.[67]

D. Io lo comprendo.

P. Ma quale secondo voi che sia maggior dolcezza tra questi due; del bacio dato o del bacio ricevuto?[68]

[57] conoscerete

[58] *ma* quello *della bocca suppera*

[59] *ancora che* fossero *posti* tutti *insieme.*

[60] Sappiate

[61] (the deleted term replaced with *è* is difficult to read, and also presents the usual addition mark)

[62] *l'una più* dolce *e più soave* dell'altra.

[63] *dici* il

[64] *che si possa sentire* nel bacio.

[65] difficoltà (the *o* corrects a *u*)

[66] *non*

[67] *Tutti gli altri baci* nelle mani (the *i* of *mani* corrects an *o*), nel *petto,* nel collo, nelle *gote, o* negli *occhi si danno;* ma *quello* solo *della bocca si dà e si riceve*

[68] *Ma* ditemi di gratia, quale credete *voi che sia maggior dolcezza;* quella *del bacio dato o del bacio ricevuto?*

D. Quanto mi può hora sovvenire, io sento maggior[e] [la] dolcezza quando la donna mia bacia me.[69]

P. Egli è in parte vero [ciò] et in parte non è vero.[70]

D. In qual maniera?[71]

P. Perché sono tre sorte baci quelli della bocca[72]: delle somme labbra, del succio, e della lingua.

D. [E]gli è vero.[73]

P. Il primo delle labbra [ugual dolcezza] porge ad ambidue, poscia che, più l'uno et l'altro [ne] dà di suo, ne riceve dall'altrui.[74] (**108v**) Et quindi è questo bacio all'uno et all'altro degli amanti meno soave degli altri due.[75]

D. È vero. Ma quale di loro sente negli altri due maggior diletto?[76]

P. Assolutamente chi[77] più ama.

D. [So] cotesto,[78] ma in caso che ambidue egualmente amino [l'un l'altro], quale di loro proverà maggior[79] dolcezza? Colui che dà o colui che riceve?

P. [In qualunque sorte {di} bacio] colui che riceve sente senza parangone maggior[80] piacere che colui che dà.

D. O cotesto, spirito mio, non ha punto[81] faccia di vero.[82]

---

[69] *Quanto a me, sento* (*a me, sento* is in fact not deleted, although Patrizi has reformulated it above) *maggior dolcezza* nell'esser baciato dalla donna mia, che nel baciare lei.

[70] Cotesto *in parte vero et in parte* è falso. (above *vero* there is an illegible deletion)

[71] E per qual cagione?

[72] Ve lo dirò, *quelli della bocca* sono tre baci

[73] *Gli è il vero.*

[74] *Il primo delle labbra porge ad ambidue* uguale dolcezza, *poscia che* né *l'uno* né *l'altro* dà del *suo* più di quello che *riceve d' altrui.*

[75] *Et quindi è* che *questo bacio all'uno et all'altro degli amanti* è *meno soave di* quello che sono *gli altri due.*

[76] Vorrei sapere *quale de'* due amanti sente maggior diletto.

[77] Quello *che*

[78] *Cotesto* io lo so

[79] più

[80] *parangone* in ogni sorte di bacio *maggior*

[81] *ponto*

[82] *verità*

P. E perché no?

D. Perché posto che in quello della lingua colui che riceve sente (come è nel vero) maggior dolcezza, che quell'altro non fa, [che dà], in tutti gli altri baci a me pare il contrario. Conciosia cosa che nel bacio del succio della bocca più dolcezza sente colui che succia, che [è] quello che dà, che non sente colui[83] che è succiato, che è colui che riceve. E così chi è baciato in[84] occhi, o in guancia, o in collo, o in petto, o in mano niuna o poca dolcezza sente, dove colui che bacia la si sente grandissima.

P. Voi argomentate il vero del bacio, [o Delfino], ma io dicevo d'un'altra cosa.

D. E di qual altra?

P. Della cagione[85] della dolcezza del bacio.

D. E quale è la cagione di questa dolcezza?[86]

P. Lo spirito dello amato, che lo amante si bee [in] baciando.

D. Cotesta sì che potrebbe bene essere qualche cosa; ma io non la intendo, [o spirito gratioso].

P. Io dico che chi bacia si bee [in]visibilmente dello spirito del baciato, et questa è la cagione onde nel bacio si senta[87] cotanta dolcezza.

D. Parte intendo e parte non intendo; là onde è mestieri che mi si faccia chiara questa cosa, che verissima[88] sembra che esser dea.

P. Vera[89] ella è per certo, ma ella non è così agevole ad ispiegarsi; per ciò che ella è di profonda contemplatione, et però vi conviene stare[90] intento molto a quello ch'io dirò.

D. Io[91] vi starò intentissimo.

P. Due cose dico io che sono quelle che cagionano nel bacio la dolcezza: l'amore, che si disse prima, e la bevuta degli spiriti dello amato, che si

---

[83] quell'altro

[84] negli

[85] *Delle cagioni*

[86] *E quale* è cotesta cagione? (Patrizi initially changed this sentence to *E quali sono coteste cagioni?* but subsequently reinstated the singular forms)

[87] *sente*

[88] bellissima

[89] Bellissima

[90] *contemplatione*, là onde se voi volete che io la vi spiani e' vi conviene *stare*

[91] Io voglio che la mi diciate, et *io*

dice hora. Per ciò che i baci che a persona non amata si danno,[92] tutto che dello spirito suo si bea, dolcezza non hanno. (**109r**) Et io mi distenderò in questo proposito a lungo, perché voi perfettamente intendiate il misterio[93] delle segrete cagioni di questa amorosa dolcezza che noi cerchiamo.

[D.] Et di questo io ti prego, o gentile spirito, che tu mi chiarisca a pieno, onde io habbia poi[94] sempre a celebrarti.

P. Statemi pur intento. Due cose habbiamo noi hora da vedere: l'una in qual modo amore faccia dolce gli spiriti dell'amato, e l'altra come essi si beano dallo[95] amante. Et dico in questa guisa, che amor nasce nei cuori humani o da simiglianza, che altri[96] habbino [in]fra di loro, o da bellezza che altri habbia in sé,[97] o da ambedue queste cose congionte. Né vi sgomenti,[98] o Delfino, a dover credere questo[99] esser vero: il vedere che donna sia radissimo ad huomo simigliante, et pure ella et ama huomo, et è da huomo amata. Per ciò che la simiglianza altra è esteriore, et altra interiore. È[100] vero che la esteriore non è cagione d'amor veruno, ma la interiore è sempre d'amor cagione. Et è ella di doppia maniera: di qualità d'animo, et di qualità di corpo. Quella del corpo è tutta nel contemperamento degli humori et degli spiriti, i quali compongono e danno vita al corpo [humano]. E quella dell'animo sta nell'impressioni che, discendendo[101] da[102] cielo, [presero dal uno stesso regnante pianeta due anime] nel loro ethereo corpicello. Quella prima corporale simiglianza è leggier cosa ad intendere, e questa seconda intenderete voi con poca[103] fatica.

---

[92] *i baci che* si danno a persona non amata (the inversion is indicated by the insertion of ·*b*· and ·*a*· above *danno* and *persona* respectively)

[93] *mistero*

[94] *per*

[95] *dello*

[96] *due*

[97] *in se stesso*

[98] (the final *i* is underlined, with an illegible deletion above)

[99] *cotesto*

[100] E

[101] *discendano*

[102] *dal*

[103] *puoca*

Et[104] dovete sapere che i pianeti operano e nei corpi elementali,[105] et in se stessi infra di loro, co'l movimento, et co'l lume recato dal movimento, co'l tepore portato dal lume, et con l'influsso delle loro proprietà dal[106] tepore trasportato. E perché il tepore et l'influsso è dal lume dependente,[107] alla variation[108] di lui prenderanno essi ancora nelle opere loro variatione, cagionata da i diversi movimenti dei cieli de' pianeti; i quali secondo che in un luogo od in altro (**109v**) del cielo si ritruovano infra di loro o più lontano, o più vicino, [o] con uno o con altro[109] aspetto si riguardano, più o meno operano, et in se stessi, e negli elementi, e negli altri corpi. Et qualhor uno di loro si ritruova, che più degli altri possa, alhora egli si dice che il dominio dell'operare è suo. Dal quale loro dominio chiunque prende impressione o qualità, o gioviale, o venereo, od[110] altro tale dal nome del regnante pianeta, si addimanda. Fino a qui credo io che voi facilmente intendiate.

D. Sì, intendo io certamente.

P. Hora mirate in questo altro canto. L'anima humana, dopo che [è] da Dio[111] creata et ha da venire a reggere corpo terreno, perché l'incorporeo, quale ella è, possa a corporeo, [quale è l'] elementale nostro corpo, [a congiungersi discendere], si veste ella un ethereo corpicello, dal quale, quasi mezano, ella è dall'uno estremo di là suso all'altro di qua giù portata, et per ciò da alcuni savii huomini vehicolo e carro dell'anima chiamato. Et in questo così fatto corpo di[112] là su di sopra i cieli l'anima, nel terreno elemento discendendo, prende [lumi et impressioni da] ciascuno de' pianeti, per le sfere de' quali ella passa[113]; ma più da quelli ne prende che più sono in forte aspetto, e più [che] di[114] tutti gli altri

---

[104] Parimenti

[105] *elementari*

[106] *del*

[107] *il tepore è l'influsso dal lume dependente*

[108] *vareation*

[109] *l'altro*

[110] *o* d'

[111] *da Dio è creata*

[112] *de*

[113] *prende ciascuno de' pianeti per le sfere de' quali ella passa* lumi et impressioni

[114] *da* (the *a* corrects an *e*; Patrizi indicates the double correction with a double underlining)

da colui il quale[115] Re [degli altri] alhora si ritruova. Da' quali[116] ella prende qualità nella maniera che altri, caminando nel sole, prende di colore fosco. Et[117] qualhora due anime [prenderanno] dal [medesimo] Regnante pianeta, o da altro di forte lume, qualità et influsso,[118] sì[119] saranno elle simiglianti,[120] et da così fatta simiglianza, o da quella del temperamento, che da questa in certa guisa si fa, et non dalla esteriore, nasce l'amore che io diceva. E se voi vedete che alcuna volta huomo[121] difforme donna[122] ami, o per contrario, donna[123] huomo sozzo, è quindi et non d'altronde. Et è (**110r**) [in] così[124] fatta maniera la somiglianza cagion dell'amore.

D. Hora intendo io et ne rimango da questo canto sodisfatto.

P. D'altro lato è la bellezza cagion più universale dell'amore, però che non è[125] bella cosa,[126] la quale non piaccia ad ogni uno.

D. Dite voi cotesto, o Patritio, o pure è l[o][127] spirito vostro che lo dice?

P. A me pare che il dica lo spirito.

D. Credete voi che gli piacesse[128] ch'io [g]li dimandassi[129] onde sia che la be[l]lezza piaccia ad ogni uno, ma però non ogni uno di[130] s[é] innamori?

---

[115] che

[116] *Dal quale*

[117] Hora

[118] *due anime dal Regnante pianeta, o da altro di forte lume, qualità et influsso* prenderanno

[119] et

[120] *simigliante*

[121] (Patrizi initially added *bell'* before *huomo*, but subsequently deleted it)

[122] *difforme* alcuna *donna*

[123] (Patrizi initially added *bella* after *donna*, but subsequently deleted it)

[124] cotesta *così* (*cotesta* was initially corrected to *questa*, which itself was then deleted)

[125] (Following *è* Patrizi made two additions that he subsequently deleted; they are illegible)

[126] *cosa* alcuna

[127] *il*

[128] *spiacesse*

[129] *dimandasse*

[130] (after *di* there is an illegible deletion which Patrizi has corrected to *lei*, itself deleted)

P. Egli mi detta ch'io vi debba rispondere che [è] di ciò[131] altissima cagione.

D. E quale è ella?

P. L'anima vostra, dice egli, anzi che del corpicello ethereo si vesta, mentre è dal suo fattore, pieno di tutte le Idee delle cose, formata, prende in sua sostanza le ragioni di[132] [tutte le] Idee. Le quali, essendo nell'Intelletto creature bellissime del più perfetto modo ch'esser[e] possano, belle ancora nell'anima si rimangono, nella più compiuta maniera che la[133] natura sua comporti.[134] Et così informata, e vestita il celeste corpicello, se ne scende per gli cieli et per gli elementi nell'alveo delle madri degli huomini, e forma l'embrione quanto può, e patisce la materia in miglior forma, corrispondente alla ragione della Idea che ella portò seco del corpo [humano]. Ogni anima dunque, che da cielo discenda, porta con esso seco la ragione della bellezza ancora e delle sue parti tutte, le quali da noi, in alcun corpo vedute e parangonate dall'anima con le ragioni, ch'ella ha in sé di loro, per lo affacimento che elle infra di loro hanno, piacciono e più e meno, secondo che minore o che maggiore affacimento l'anima vi conosce. E conciosia cosa che ogni anima humana ha cotali ragioni in sé di bellezza, et ogni una, per certo rammentamento di loro, può delle bellezze corporali fare alle sue incorporali parangone, [è] di qui[135] (**110v**) che ad ogni uno piacciono[136] le bellezze e le sue parti; le quali sono: le proportioni delle parti corporali, i lineamenti, i colori, i lumi, l'ombre, e le gratie, le quali, e tutte insieme e ciascuna per sé stessa, piacciono.[137] Ma come fanno innamorare? direte voi. Et non ogni uno?

D. Cotesto è quello che io cerco.

P. A cotesto io dico che altra cosa è piacimento,[138] altra desiderio, altra affettione, et altra amore. Piacimento è un godimento dell'animo in[139] se

---

[131] *di ciò* n'è

[132] *d*elle

[133] nel*la*

[134] patisca

[135] *qui* nasce

[136] *piaccceno*

[137] *piaccceno*

[138] *piaccimento*

[139] di

stesso, [in] contemplando veduta bellezza, od[140] altra buona o perfetta cosa. Ma desiderio è uno appetito di possedere la piacciuta; e l'affettione è un[a] inclinatione di giovare alla medesima; et Amore è un composto int[i]ero di piacimento, di desiderio, e di affetione. Hora[141] io dico in questa guisa, che ogni bellezza piace ad ogni uno, dopo il quale piacimento non è huomo alcuno che non desideri di possederla. Ma non è già che ogni huomo habbia inclinatione di giovare alla piaciuta e desiderata cosa. Il che io dissi affettione, la quale, tantosto che è al piacimento et al desiderio aggionta, se ne fa l'amore, ma senza lei non[142] si può [egli] già fare. Hora questa affettione per certo non nasce da bellezza, poscia che ogni bellezza piacendo e facendo di sé desiderio non fa innamorare, ma nasce bene ella dalla predetta occulta simiglianza, poscia ch'ei si vede ch'huom, incontrando tal hora persona né bella[143] né gratiosa, è da occulta cagione tirato porle affettione. La qual cagione altro non è che quella simiglianza che dicemmo, o dell'animo[144] o del corpo. Hora, così come la bellezza può in persona ritrovarsi la quale a noi non sia simile, così può la simiglianza altresì in persona ritrovarsi[145] la quale bella non sia. Et per ciò per la primiera si farà in noi piacimento e desiderio, et per la seconda affettione, ma appartato[146] ciascheduno, sì come congionti (111r) insieme tutti si farà[147] in noi amore, qualhor bellezza e simiglianza di noi in una stessa persona se ritruovi. Il concorso adunque di[148] piacimento, di[149] desiderio, et di[150] affettione è veramente l'amore. Et quindi è che ogni bellezza faccia piacimento et desiderio di sé in ogni uno, et

---

[140] *o* d'

[141] (Patrizi corrects the *h* to a capital)

[142] *lei* egli *non*

[143] *né* di *bella*

[144] (The *o* is emphasised by Patrizi)

[145] ritrovarsi in persona (the inversion is indicated with the insertion of ·*b*· and ·*a*· above *ritrovarsi* and *persona* respectively)

[146] *Affettione*, anco apparato (Patrizi initially attempts to correct *apparato* to *appartato* within the original word, but subsequently deletes it and adds the correction above)

[147] *tutti* se faranno

[148] *d*el

[149] *d*el

[150] *d*ell'

non però di sé ogni uno innamori[151]; et [è] anco chiaro quale bellezza sia quell'altra che faccia gli huomini l'un dell'altro innamorare, et perché[152] tal hora bell'huomo ami[153] men bella donna, et bella donna men bello huomo.

D. Sì cotesto[154]; ma egli non è già chiaro, o spirito gratioso e pien d'amore, onde sia che bella donna ami tal hor sozzo huomo, e bello huomo difforme donna.

P. Cotesto sarà anco chiaro se voi considererete che amore altro sia brutto e[t] ferino amore, et altro amore bello et degno di huomo[155]; de' quali[156] l'uno è tutto alla bruttura della lusuria inchinato, et l'altro quasi tutto è dato al godimento del conversare e dell'amare bellamente.

D. Cotesto è ben[e] vero, ma che fa egli in pro del mio quesito?

P. Fa egli che quell'amore, che è da sozzo a sozzo e da bello a sozzo, è ferino e[t] brutto[157] [amore sempre], et a fine di solo sfogamento de' focosi appetiti di brutta anima. [Ma] quello che è da deforme a bello, e da bello a bello, è il più et di propria natura [della bella maniera d'amore. Et può quindi essere] {che} le due prime maniere d'amore non nascano da simiglianza. Ma da bellezza non nascono elle già mai per certo, e però elle sono [maniere] imperfettissime [d'amore]. Ma le due seconde sempre et da simiglianza et da bellezza nasceranno, et però sono elle sempre d'amore perfette et compiute maniere.[158]

D. Hora resto io della seconda mia questione pago e sodisfatto, et però ritorna, o spirito amoroso e pien di gentilezza, ad ispedire la prima della dolcezza de' baci. (**111v**)

P. Io sono contento [di così fare], ma voi attendetemi con intentione. Nascendo le belle e perfette maniere d'amore da simiglianza e da bellezza,

---

[151] s'*innamori*

[152] *per ciò* (before *per* is an addition that was subsequently deleted and is now illegible)

[153] *am*a

[154] *cotest*a

[155] *considererete che* due sorti d'*amore* si trovano: l'uno è *brutto e ferino,* et l'*altro* è *bello et degno di huomo*

[156] *de*i *quali* amori *l'uno*

[157] *è* sempre *ferino e brutto, et a fine*

[158] *da bello a bello,* per *il più è di propria natura* (Patrizi has added and subsequently deleted) *d'huomo*). *Le due prime maniere* non possono nascere già mai d'amore, *e però elle sono imperfettissime*. Quelle altre due, perché nascono da simiglianza e da bellezza sono perfette e compiute, e sempre causano amore.

et in loro per lor natura sentendosi perfetta la dolcezza de' baci, la quale dissi[159] io esservi entro[160] da amore sparsa, egli è da vedere in qual maniera amore la vi sparga [entro la dolcezza], e come per questo mezo siano i baci così soave cosa. Sopra a che ragionando, io farò mio principal ragionamento in su'l più nobile et in su'l più bell'amore di tutti gli altri, nel quale è veramente la perfetta dolcezza del bacio.

D. Sì, è vero; ma ella non è però così sua, [o gentile spirito], che non vi habbia parte [anco] quello altro, che men bell'amore[161] [è].

P. Egli è vero cotesto. Ma è ciò per accidente, non per natura, conciosia cosa che quella rabbia focosa, che ha huom in quell'amore, fa quel dolce parer[e] che non è. Et è quella dolcezza di imaginatione [più tosto] e di inganno, che di verità,[162] di che non è in proposito nostro di ragionare.

D. Se [e]gli è così, o spirito pien di bontà e di virtù, [et tu] lascia di parlar[e] di questa, e segui della vera e della natural dolcezza del bacio.

P. Così farò. Ma voi [mi] dite,[163] sapete [voi] quale sia la guida che conduca amore ne' cuori humani?

D. Io non intendo che sia altro che la simiglianza già detta e la bellezza.[164]

P. Coteste sono le genitrici e le madri dell'amore, ma io dimando quale sia il Duce, che nell'human cuore dalla[165] simiglianza e dalla[166] bellezza conduce amore.

D. Cotesto non so io.

P. Gli occhi, che[167] sono essi altro che un varco, per lo quale amore dal bello simile nella vostra anima, o huomini, si tragitta.[168]

---

[159] *disse*

[160] *dentro*

[161] *habbia* anco *parte quella altra, che è men bell'amare.*

[162] *rabbia focosa, che* fa *in quell'amore parer* dolce al huomo quello *che non è* una *dolcezza,* che nasce più tosto *da imaginatione e da inganno, che da verità*

[163] *voi dite*mi

[164] *simiglianza* e la bellezza già detta. (the inversion is indicated by the insertion of *b·* and *·a·* above *bellezza* and *già* respectively, and further emphasised with two addition marks)

[165] *della*

[166] *della*

[167] *non*

[168] *tragetta*

D. E per qual modo si tragitta[169] egli per quindi, o spirito amoroso[?]

P. Non per altro che perché i raggi degli occhi (**112r**) e de' lumi di tutta la bellezza[170] del bello simile portano con esso seco degli spiriti del cuore di lui. E, con uno affisarsi[171] negli occhi vostri, gittano[172] per quindi se stessi[173] nel vostro cuore, et della[174] bellezza, donde escono essi, gli spiriti di lui stampando, l'accendono anco con le lor fiamme. E questi[175] sono i veri dardi, e le saette, e le facelle d'Amore, con le quali, saettando egli et infiammando i cuori altrui, vi fa entro quelle piaghe così dolci e quelle fiamme così ardenti, le quali, per quantunque gran dolcezza che si bea poi,[176] non si risanano o si ristringnono.[177] [E stato siete voi mai, o amoroso] Delfino, arso[178] di così fatto amore?

D. Sì, sono io per certo, [o spirito gentile, acceso] hora di così fatto.[179] Ma vorrei io che tu più a lungo mi dichiarassi questo tragitto de' raggi e degli spiriti altrui nel nostro cuore.

P. Io il[180] farò volontieri. [La prima cosa] voi [e'] dovete sapere che generalmente in tutti gli occhi e[t][181] molta diversità de' colori, [o] molta di chiarezza, e[t] molta di copia di spiriti e di raggi [si ritruova]. [Ma non ne si ha niuno il quale tanto habbia di spiriti e di raggi[182]], et per ciò di splendore, quanto n'ha quello che communemente da voi si dice occhio allegro, e che per ciò più faccia altrui innamorare, che si faccia egli. Et è l'occhio allegro di due colori e non di più: nero, et azuro, che bianco

---

[169] *tragetta*

[170] *bellezza e del*

[171] *affissarsi*

[172] *gettano*

[173] *stesso*

[174] *dalla* (the *a* is traced by Patrizi)

[175] (the *i* is traced by Patrizi)

[176] (the word was initially deleted by Patrizi and subsequently rewritten)

[177] *ristringono*

[178] O (here, an illegible mark and question mark have been deleted) *Delfino,* siete voi mai *arso*

[179] *per certo,* et *hora di così fatto* fuoco mi consumo

[180] *lo*

[181] *è*

[182] (after *raggi* Patrizi inserted *et per ciò*, before subsequently deleting it to avoid repetition)

dice il volgo. Per ciò che gli altri di mezo, o non sono occhi allegri, o tanto sono quanto hanno o dell'uno o dell'altro dei due colori nominati, de' quali il nero, con lo paragone che fa con la bianchezza della carne dell'occhio, fa più bella vista senza dubbio, et è più bello communemente giudicato. Ma l'azuro nel vero fa altrui più tosto innamorare; e ciò non per altro è che per la copia degli spiriti e di raggi, li quali sono le vere saette di amore, e la facella, con le quali egli fere et incende invisibilmente l'anime[183] altrui.

D. Cotesta cosa io la credo, (**112v**) [gentile spirito, essere vera], ma, perché io ne sia capace,[184] ella ha mistieri di più aperto dimostramento.

P. Et io non mi stancherò[185] in tutto hoggi in[186] farvi pago de' tutte le quistioni vostre,[187] pure che voi mi ascoltiate.

D. [Et] io non mi stancherò in cento anni d'ascoltarti, o gentile e nobile spirito, né tu mi puoi dare più soave né più gradito nutrimento di questo che mi dai, di che io mi te ne terrò in eterno tenuto.[188]

P. Ascoltatemi adunque intentamente. Tutte le cose operate dalla madre natura, perché hebbero nel loro generamento per padre il sole, ritennero ciascuna, secondo il lor potere, delle paterne qualità, conciosia cosa che di loro altre ritennero di luce, altre di colore, che[189] lume [è] di materia vestito,[190] et altre ritennero insieme e di luce e di colore. Così fatte sono le pretiose pietre il più, e gli occhi delli animali, i quali e colore hanno e luce. E conciosia cosa che ogni corpo, c'habbia luce, sparga dalla[191] sua luce raggi, i quali portino con esso loro lume da illuminare intorno a loro l'aere oscuro, hanno e[t] le pietre predette, e gli occhi delli animali, et dell'huomo e luce e raggi. Di questo non dovete [voi], o Delfino, portar dubbio veruno, conciosia cosa che si vegga[no] notturni ucelli et animali havere la notte occhi chiari e risplendenti; il che, quantunque non

---

[183] *anima*

[184] meglio *capace*

[185] satierò

[186] per

[187] *de* vostri desiderii

[188] obligato

[189] *che è lume*

[190] (Patrizi has marked this sentence with two vertical lines, one each at the beginning and end)

[191] *d*ella (the *a* is traced by Patrizi)

si vegga così chiaro negli occhi vostri, egli è però vero che sieno luminosi. Per ciò che, s'altri con dito calcherà il canto dell'occhio verso il naso, vi ci vederà[192] entro chiaro un circoletto pien di lume, il qual[e] è certo argumento della luce de' vostri occhi, la qual[193] così in voi huomini, come anco negli animali antedetti, manda raggi di sé; il che l'esperienza vi dimostra palese. Per ciò che quelli animali ch'io dissi veggono nella notte chiaramente, la qual cosa esser[e] non potrebbe in verun modo se i raggi de' proprii occhi loro non illuminassero d'intorno l'aere tenebroso, et voi non potreste vedere lo splendore degli occhi loro se egli da' raggi loro (113r) non fusse a gli occhi vostri trasportato. Di che non è alcuna più forte prova che se tengono gli animali [predetti] gli occhi fissi in terra, o in altra cosa soda e tersa, vi si forma all'incontro degli occhi loro un picciolo cerchietto luminoso, corrispondente alla puppilla de' loro occhi, la qual cosa da altro non può esser già che venga che da i raggi degli occhi, i quali portano la luce degli occhi a terminare là dove essi hanno finimento. È anco il medesimo negli[194] occhi humani, per ciò che io so che Mario nella carcere, essendo in luoco oscuro, ispaventò col lume degli occhi suoi colui che era stato [da Silla] ad ucciderlo mandato. Et Tiberio, destatosi la notte in istanza tenebrosa, vedea per alquanta pezza tutto ciò che vi era; il che per altro essere non può che avvenisse se non perché i raggi degli occhi portassero il lume per quel tempo con esso seco. Et Augusto haveva i raggi visivi così forti e così pieni di luce, che, s'egli mirava fisso negli occhi altrui, quasi abbagliando[gli] a volgersi altrove [g]li constringeva; la qual cosa per altro [essere] non pare[195] se non perché il troppo lume de' suoi rifrangeva i raggi degli altrui, e sforzavali a fugire quello incontro. Da queste tante e così forti[196] pr[u]ove, io credo, o Delfino, che voi crediate che gli occhi humani habbiano in sé luce, e che essi da sé mandino raggi luminosi.

D. Io credo senza dubbio che così sia.

---

[192] (between the *v* and *e* Patrizi has deleted a now-illegible letter)

[193] (Patrizi added, and subsequently deleted, *anco*)

[194] *degli*

[195] *per altro non p*uote essere *se*

[196] *forte*

P. Io dico [adunque] hora degli spiriti, i quali furno l'altra qualità degli occhi innamoranti, et incommincierommi[197] di qui. Lo spirito, prendendolo in human significato, altro non è che un vapore sottilissimo di sangue, generato nel cuore dal natural calore di lui, il quale spirito per sue vene, che i medici addimandano arterie, porta il caldo del cuore per tutte in sino le minute particelle[198] del vivente corpo, le quali tutte egli conserva e calde e vive. Et è vero operatore del calore e della vita altrui, et conciosia che ogni calda cosa[199] e[t] (113v) sottile per sua natura saglia allo[200] in su, molta parte dello spirito, che tale è, saglie dal cuore al capo et al cervello, et quivi, dalla temperatura di lui più che prima purificato, si fa stormento non[201] della vita [più] ma delle conoscenti potenze dell'anima e de' movimenti corporali. Per ciò che egli per disposti vasi è dalla natura mandato a gli stormenti del sentire et della volontà, et a i nervi movitori, donde l'huomo si move e sente. Quivi due vasi in guisa di due vene partono da i ventricelli del cervello a gli occhi, e portano[202] lo spirito [quivi] purgato a loro. E perché essi sono ampii assai, corre anco lo spirito per loro a gli occhi [assai] abondante,[203] il quale, per ciò che da se stesso è chiaro, mischiando la sua chiarezza con la naturale chiarezza degli occhi, fa negli animali e nell'huomo chiara e risplendente questa parte, più che tutte le altre parti.

D. Si vede egli bene, o spirito gentile, che gli occhi sono la più chiara parte di tutte l'altre. Ma che argomento hai tu che lo spirito aggiunga loro chiarezza?

P. Chiaro argomento ne è la ragione de' corpi caldi e sottili, i quali tutti hanno chiarezza, et oltra ne fa la sperienza un altro; per ciò che chiara cosa [è] che l'occhio del huomo vivo è più chiaro assai che non è quello dell'huom[204] morto. Di che non è altra cosa cagione che perché egli ha di più del morto lo spirito, il che vi conferma ancora un altro caso, e

[197] *incommincieremo*

[198] *per tutte* le parti *del*

[199] *ogni* cosa calda (the inversion is indicated by the insertion of ·b· and ·a· above *cosa* and *calda* respectively)

[200] *alto*

[201] *non* più *della*

[202] *portano* quivi *lo*

[203] *abondante*mente

[204] *huomo*

ciò è quando la pupilla dell'occhio è maggiore egli è più risplendente che quando ella è, per alcuna fatica, minore; et ciò è perché, consumandosi nella fatica gli spiriti del capo, essi non corrono a gli occhi così copiosi.

D. Di tanto io resto pago, spirito gratioso.

P. Lo spirito adunque, venendo alla stremità di tutto'l corpo, e spinto dal battimento del cuore e dal movimento delle membra per quei piccioli apparenti e nascosti pertugietti della pelle, i quali voi huomini addimandate[205] pori, se n'esce fuori e si disperde. Et il medesimo fa egli per li medesimi pertugietti degli occhi, i quali quivi son parimente, sì come sono per tutto il vostro corpo. Per li quali pertugietti uscendo lo spirito, (**114r**) agevolmente, sì come co' suoi simili, si congiunge et si unisce co' raggi degli occhi, e con loro si discorre sino a tanto che, contrastando la forza sua con le forze di fuori, in essere il mantiene. Ma tosto che egli è dalle nimiche forze[206] estinto, il raggio si riman vedovo di lui.

D. Cotesto va bene, spirito buono et intendente; ma da che mi provi tu questa unione dello spirito e del raggio, e per ciò che a me sembra difficile molto?

P. Da due prove manifesto il provo io, l'una delle quali è quella che si vede in donna nei tempi dei suoi sangui, la quale, mirando nel[lo] specchio, il macchia quasi di gocciole sanguigne, il che altro non è che perché lo spirito, il quale humido di quei sangui e dal raggio portato al piano dello specchio, et quivi per lo freddo di lui agghiacciando, ghiocciola diviene.

D. S'ella è vera, cotesta è grande isperienza.

P. Voi nela[207] potete sempre a vostro diletto provare. Ma l'ho io più volte da un filosofo spirito mio amico inteso, che egli ad Aristotile il dimostrò, il quale poi ne' suoi libri lo scrisse. Ma l'altra prova si è che, s'altri mira fiso per alquanto spatio negli occhi infermi d'altrui, egli de' suoi medesimamente inferma; la qual cosa vi fo fede io essere al vostro Petrarca avvenuto dal destro occhio della sua Laura. Il che anco so che egli scrisse nelle sue amorose passioni, et voi giovani innamorati vel dovreste[208] sapere.

---

[205] *i quali* s'*addimanda*no
[206] cose
[207] *nella*
[208] *dovrest*i

D. Sì,[209] egli è in quel[210] sonetto: Qual ventura mi fu quando dall'uno.
P. E questa cosa per certo non è per incanto o per malia, ma è virtù
naturale, et la natura non opera gli effetti suoi se non per alcun mezo, e,
tra l'occhio di lei e quello di lui, io so che altro mezo che dagli occhi loro
uscisse non fu che il raggio e lo spirito di che vi ragiono, e so che fu lo
spirito quello che quella infermità recò nell'occhio del Petrarca. Ma noi
siamo giunti hoggimai a quel passo per lo quale nell'anima vostra passa
amore, e però egli vi convien stare intentissimo, [o Delfino].
D. Io ci starò intentissimo.
P. Uscendo lo spirito dall'un occhio insieme col raggio luminoso, viene a
ritrovare l'occhio altrui. Quivi, se l'uno e l'altro di loro dell'un occhio è
[molto e] chiaro molto più dell'altro, lo sforza et abbaglia, nel modo
che Augusto abbagliava[211] gli occhi altrui. Et abbagliandolo, fatti più
larghi i pori suoi et aumentato lo spirito dalla forza dello (114v) affissamento, penetra dentro a loro, e ritrovando [esso] gli spiriti di là entro
non nemici, ma quasi fratelli e sotto il medesimo dominio nati, si mischia
con esso loro volontieri, in compagnia de' quali, sì come sottili, va diritto
a ritrovare il cuore, dal quale sono quegli altri nati, sì come a luogo
naturalmente caro et conservatore. Così portato lo spirito forastiero dal
famigliare al cuore, e con la sottilità sua penetrando per entro la sostanza
di lui, più che egli non era prima l'infiamma; et per la dimestichezza
presa per la simiglianza che egli ha con li spiriti di lui famigliari, quasi
in proprio luogo venuto, il si fa volontieri albergo. Et il cuore, che si
truova nuovo hoste havere, sì perché egli è per sé dolce et sì perché
viene da cuor simile et non odioso, ha cara la sua venuta et il ritiene
volontieri. Cotesta è filosofia, o Delfino, non già da altri che da intel-
letti innamorati. Ma oltre, [conciosia cosa] che nell'entrata che fece[212]
lo spirito forestiero per gli occhi, con esso seco vi entra anco la imagine
della bellezza donde ei deriva, egli si forma gli spiriti del cuore albergatore di quella forma che è [la] bellezza, che egli là entro portò con

---

[209] Se
[210] quell
[211] abbagliò
[212] fa

esso seco. La quale poi l'anima ragionevole, negli[213] spiriti veggendo[214] et riconoscendola in gran parte simile alla ragione che ella ha in sé della bellezza del corpo humano, la parangona con essa la ragione; nel qual paraggio sempre avviene che l'anima contemplatrice, dalla maraviglia di quella bellezza e dall'amorevolezza di quella somiglianza ingannando sé medesima, aggiunga[215] a' deffetti della bellezza le perfettioni della ragion[e] sua. Dal qual inganno nasce poi quello inganno commune degli amanti, che più bella sempre stimano[216] la bellezza amata, che ella non è nel vero. Così fatto è adunque, o Delfino amoroso, il modo col quale amore ha entrata ne' vostri cuori; et dal caldo et dalla simiglianza degli spiriti forestieri entrati, sono quelle fiamme et quella dolcezza che si sente nel cuore l'huomo innamorato. Et in questo modo fa amore gli spiriti dello amato dolci e soavi, poscia che per lo mezo di loro (**115r**) egli ha quegli dell'amante raddolciti e fatti a quegli dell'amato simiglianti.

D. Belli e maravigliosi segreti mi hai tu, amorosissimo spirito, fatto palesi.[217] Ma tu mi di' ancora, io te ne priego, virtuosissimo spirito, in qual modo è che lo affissamento degli occhi luminosi e belli della donna ha forza di far passare gli spiriti suoi ne' cuori altrui et accendervi amore, et non hanno così forza quegli dell'huomo, quantunque luminosi, di far passare nel cuore della donna gli spiriti suoi, et farla altresì di sé[218] innamorare?

P. Già vi ho detto io, [o Delfino], che [se] lo spirito non è chiaro molto e copioso, onde abbagliando apra i pori dell'occhio altrui et entro vi entri, non ha potere di accendere in alcun cuore fiamma amorosa. Là onde molto di rado[219] si vedrà, o non mai, che altri s'innamori di questo amore, se non per lo mezo di occhi chiari e risplendenti. Per la qual cosa, se la donna per caso s'avviene in occhi di giovane huomo luminosi et di spirito ripieni, indrizzati fisamente ne' suoi, così si resta ella accesa di lui come egli di lei, et quindi sono e non d'altronde le vicendevoli fiamme in

---

[213] *nelli*
[214] *veggendo*la
[215] *aggiunge*
[216] *estimano*
[217] *palese*
[218] *s'*
[219] *raro*

amore. Et in caso che gli occhi del giovine huomo non sieno molto luminosi, e per ciò non sieno possenti ad infiammar lei, si resta ella nondimeno
con affettione amorosa verso di lui, per quella simiglianza che è tra loro,
quantunque ella infiamata affatto, per non haver[e] quel dardo ricevuto
che egli, non rimanga. Et di qui sì vi voglio accertar io, o Delfino, che
non è donna la quale faccia altrui di sé innamorare giamai che, o parimente ella non venga presa d'amore, o che ella non si resti almeno verso
l'innamorato affettionata. Per la qual cosa dovete voi più volontieri amar
sempre, poscia che voi siete sicuro che voi ne siete, o del pari,[220] o di
poco men ricambiato.

D. Cotesta così buona novella, se la sapessero gli amanti, o spirito gentilis-
simo, molte gratie ti renderebbono; et io per me la dirò a quantunque[221]
n'incontro (**115v**), perché te ne sieno eternamente tenuti.

P. Et così fate, o Delfino,[222] ma seguiamo più avanti. Rimanendo l'anima
stampata dalla[223] bellezza altrui, si conserva ella per gran tempo quella
imagine intera[224] e salda. Ma gli spiriti, secondo che sono sostanze
sottili et che nella continua fatica del cuore si vanno disperdendo, rimasi
privi della soavità del caldo altrui et della dolcezza della compagnia, del
continuo van desiderando rinovamento[225] di sé medesimi, e nuovo ricevimento de' loro fratei carnali. Et quindi nasce l'ardentissimo desiderio di
rivedere gli occhi innamora[n]ti, ne' quali mirando il Petrarca io so che
sentì tanta dolcezza che stimò nulla tutte l'altre dolcezze degli amanti.
[Così adunque si desidera dagli amanti] il revidimento della persona
amata, e degli occhi specialmente, per lo rinovamento delle proprie
fiamme e della dolcezza, che il cuor[e] prova dalla compagnia del suo
hoste. Ma donde è, direte voi, il desiderio del toccare l'amato? E la
dolcezza del baciare? Che fu, o Delfino, la vostra principal questione.

D. Così fu, gentile spirito, et a questa scendi hoggimai.

P. Vi rispondo io che egli per altra cagione non è che per cagione del
medesimo rinovamento dello ardore e della gioia del cuore. Il che si

---

[220] *peri*

[221] quanti (Patrizi attempted to modify the end of the word, adding *tunque*, then
deleted it altogether and rewrote it below, probably because the original was illegible)

[222] Vi ringratio, *ma*

[223] *dalla* sua

[224] *intiera*

[225] ritro*vamento*

fa in questa guisa: il cuore, il quale per sua natura ha movimento di ristringersi e d'allargarsi, nello allargamento che egli fa, tira l'aere in sé da' polmoni, che il tirano dal naso e dalla bocca, e tira anco l'aere da tutta la circonferenza della pelle per que' pertugetti nominati pori, a i quali finiscono insensibili arterie, ch'io dissi vasi e canali degli spiriti. Per lo contrario, nel ristringimento che il cuore fa di sé, egli si vuota degli spiriti e dell'aere tirato, et vuotandosi per lo sospingimento delle parti, corrono per le arterie gli spiriti impulsi fino alla bocca loro, finiente nella pelle, (116r) et per i pertugetti già detti s'escono del corpo. Et questo di continuo fa il cuore, mentre e' vive, per rinovamento e per rifrescamento degli spiriti suoi e del suo calore, da che è il mantenimento della sua vita. Attendete hora al passo, o Delfino. Il cuore innamorato, secondo cuore, desidera rinovamento de' suoi spiriti, ma, secondo cuore innamorato, desidera [rinovamento] della sua gioia,[226] la quale dal[227] disperdimento di quei spiriti, che la gli facevano, si sciema et manca; et puotegli esser rinovata da spiriti fratelli de' primieri, e ciò li può venire o per riveduta degli occhi amati o a[228] più copia per toccamento della persona amata. Perciò che nel toccamento di lei avviene che, tirando il cuore innamorato con moto naturale per via dell'arterie l'aria, in luogo di lei ritrovando gli spiriti dell'amato, per la medesima via mandati fuora dal cuore di lui, tira loro in vece dell'aria e soavemente se ne ristora; onde egli sente e fiamme e dolcezze rinovate. La qual cosa che vera sia due certissimi argomenti vi recherò [io]. L'uno de' quali è questo: che con quanta più parte del suo corpo l'amante tocca il corpo dell'amato, tanto più et ardore[229] et gioia sente; et con quanta per contrario meno, meno. E[t è] ciò a ragione, perciò che all'hora per più arterie tira in sé gli spiriti dello amato, et hora ne gli tira per meno, e meno copia ne riceve. L'altra pruova è che, se per alcun caso il corpo dello amato è freddo all'hora che l'amante il tocca, egli sente o poca o niuna dolcezza o fuoco; et è ciò perché il freddo per sua natura costringe i pori in guisa che gli spiriti dell'amato non ne possono[230] uscire, e per conseguente non gli possono i pori dell'amante in sé tirare. Et, se volete, vi può per terza pruova venire

---

[226] *gioia* rinovamento
[227] *dal*lo
[228] da *più*
[229] *arde*
[230] *possano*

che più dolcezza oltre modo sente l'amante nello stringersi[231] la cosa amata, che nel toccarla simplicemente non sente. La qual cosa è perché in (**116v**) quello stringimento si affanna alquanto e l'uno e l'altro cuore, onde sono sforzati amendui a mandare et a tirare con più forza gli spiriti dell'altro et a più copia; donde nasce che quelli, da sé mandando a più copia [et questi a più copia dall'altro tirando, a più copia sente et dolcezza et ardore].[232] Ma vengo hora al bacio. Egli[233] non è per altro dolce [il bacio] all'innamorato che perché egli tira in sé et bee degli spiriti dell'amato, bacisi egli o mano, o petto, o collo, o guancia, od occhi, o bocca. Per la qual stessa cagione il bacio del succio è più dolce che non è quello delle sopreme labbra, perciò che non solo egli si raccoglie quelli che sono del cuore amato mandati fuora, ma con la forza del tiro se ne tira egli degli[234] altri a forza, e tutti se gli bee. D'onde anco è che più degli altri succi[235] è dolce il succio della bocca, perché per quindi, come per più larga via, molti più ne tira, che per quei piccioli pertugietti della pelle. D[i] questo bacio del succio è anco più dolce il bacio della lingua, conciosia cosa che egli non solo tira quella medesima copia degli spiriti che'l succio,[236] ma la si[237] tira egli molto maggiore di lui,[238] perciò che egli si tiri[239] quelli della lingua ancora, la quale è tutta spongioso corpo et n'è del continuo ripiena, et anco gusta dell'interior humore del corpo amato. Il quale humore ha caldo e spiriti insieme misti; le quali due dolcezze congiunte et miste insieme dell'humore e degli spiriti copiosi, tirati dal cuore amato, cagionano quei battimenti, quegli illanguidimenti, e quegli sfinimenti di lui, che ammortiscono e fanno in un tratto immobili et insensati i corpi altrui.

D. Hora sono io pago, et hora sono io del tutto contento, et hora intendo, mercé tua, o cortesissimo spirito, queste alte maraviglie e questi

---

[231] *stringere*

[232] (*sente e dolcezza et ardore* was in fact already present in the original text; Patrizi evidently added it in error, and then neglected to delete it)

[233] (Patrizi corrects the *e* to a capital)

[234] *delli*

[235] (Patrizi traces the upper part of the *c*)

[236] *succio* suol tirare

[237] se ne

[238] *maggiore* copia;

[239] *tira*

dolcissimi segreti.[240] Ma dimmi, per finimento d'ogni cosa, o spirito amorosissimo, donde è quel bacio della morditura, et donde è anco che si bacino quell'altre parti[241] da te ricordate?

P. Il mordimento fa l'innamorato non(**117r**) per tirare più spiriti in sé di quello che si faccia per lo succio, ma perché, raccordatosi che egli arde per quella persona, et è da lei nel cuore offeso, spinto[242] da un subbito desiderio di vendetta in quella che [la] possiede, adopra quelle armi che più preste gli sono. Ma ricordatosi che egli ha anco vita per lei, prestamente pentito volge quella vendetta in dolce nutrimento delle sue fiamme. Si[243] baciano le mani come quelle che sono ministre de' pensieri dell'amato cuore. Il petto si bacia come albergo di loro. Ma il collo donde porga tanta dolcezza nel bacio suo, non vuole Amore, o Delfino, che [io] vi[244] scuopra al presente. Ma pregatenel divotamente che, nell'avvenire almeno, egli si degni di scoprirvi e questo et un altro segreto del medesimo bacio; il quale è che molto maggior dolcezza si sente baciando nella sinistra parte del collo, che nella destra. [Ma] la guancia si bacia come più vero e più proprio albergo della bellezza del viso, perciò che ella è propria sede de' colori[245] che la fanno e della vivacità de' lumi. Gli occhi si baciano come primiera e potentissima cagione delle fiamme e delle gioie altrui. La bocca ultimamente si bacia perché ella è bocca dell'anima e del cuore, e canale più ampio degli spiriti dell'amato, e più che ogni altro copiosa et abbondante. [Et è] il bacio del petto[246] più dolce di quello delle mani, perché gli spiriti che quindi si beono vengono più di vicino e più nuovi dal cuore produttore. Quella delle guancie è dolcezza in parte dell'opinione dell'amante, il quale si crede di bersi quindi tutta et intiera la bellezza amata. La[247] cagione del bacio e la dolcezza del bacio della bocca havete voi già inteso a pieno. Quella degli occhi a ragione avanza la dolcezza dell'altre parti, fuor che

---

[240] *secreti*

[241] *parte*

[242] *spirito*

[243] (Patrizi corrects the *s* to a capital)

[244] *vi* lo

[245] *coloro*

[246] (*petto* is followed by *è* in the original text, which Patrizi probably forgot to delete)

[247] (Patrizi corrects the *l* to a capital)

de[248] la bocca, perciò che l'amante ferito dalle saette loro dolcissime e soavi, baciando loro, consola le sue piaghe et bee con nuovi spiriti nuova dolcezza. Ma quella del collo non vuole Amore che io vi dimostri, infino che voi non gli havete offerto sacrificio degno di lui.

D. Et quale sacrificio gli si conviene, o spirito amoroso e buono? Ma egli non risponde, o Patritio.

P. Certamente egli non parlerà più, perciò che egli dee haver adempito le vostre dimande.

D. O Amore potentissimo Dio, io ti ringratio con tutta l'anima, poiché ti sei degnato hoggi di palesarmi tanti tuoi maravigliosi segreti, in cognition de' quali [così alta] non è per ancora pervenuto huomo alcuno. (**117v**) Io ti sacrifico questa anima e questo cuore, se essi sono però hostie degne della tua deità, e se non sono ti prego divotamente che tu mi discuopra quale holocausto ti diletti, perché io possa alla tua deità per tanti benefici, et hoggi et sempre da te ricevuti, grato dimostrarmi. Di questo ti supplico, perché, mancando io del debito mio, non provochi l'ira tua contra di me, al quale tu sia sempre propitio e favorevole.

>Vidi Amor, che nel bel candido seno
>>Del'Idol mio, que' dolci spirti cari
>>Giva pascendo, e con soavi avari
>>Baci fea[249] sé di lor dolcezza pieno.
>L'alma, che dell'invidia venia meno,
>>Là corse, e i be' celesti spirti chiari
>>Famelica sen gio,[250] d'Amor al pari,
>>Beendo, e non fia mai ber satia a pieno.
>Amor, che di sì dolce vita privo
>>Si vide,[251] con l'ardente face l'arse
>>L'ali, e più far non puote a me ritorno.
>Idolo mio, perch'io ti torni vivo,
>>Lascia, ti prego, con le labbra scarse
>>Ch'io l'alma colga al tuo bel sen intorno.

---

[248] *di*

[249] *fra*

[250] *gia*

[251] *vede*

(106r) The Delfino, or the Kiss

Dialogue of Francesco Patrizio. Interlocutors: Delfino[i] and Patrizio.

DEL. I have come to find you so that you might free me of a thought from which I am unable to free myself. It is one that seems to me very difficult and entirely novel.[ii]

PATR. Welcome, my dear Mr. Angelo. But what is this thought that is causing you such trouble?

DEL. Many times I have pondered the great sweetness that is found in the kiss; which truly is so great that even if it is not the first among of love's pleasures, it is certainly the second. And many times I have sought the cause of this, without ever being able to establish it to my satisfaction, such that my mind should find peace. I have also turned to those writers who write about love, and in them I truly find many beautiful and marvellous things; but nothing about the kiss, as if it had no force or value in love.[iii] For this reason I decided to come to you, so that you might reveal to me why it is that the kiss is so sweet.

PATR. You have given yourself poor counsel, Mr. Angelo Amoroso, that you should come to a hermit[iv] with questions about love, and one intent on other studies; for you know that the hermitage is no place for the study of love.

DEL. My counsel was good, for I know that before you became a hermit you were in love[v]; and I also know that you already understand, both by proof[vi] and by learning, what love is. Therefore, prepare yourself to answer my question.

PATR. All of a sudden you wish for me to explain a subject of magnitude, and one so novel, without my knowing what I should say or think.

DEL. It is certainly much easier for you to give some answer to my question than for me to return on another occasion (106v), and by so harsh a road. Therefore, I ask you to take a little trouble in order to save me the great trouble of returning up this arduous slope, and I shall be all the more indebted to you.

PATR. You rouse me, dear Mr. Angelo, with these words; and now I see that you must be a great sorcerer, for your pleas have the force to dispose my mind to speak of things of which I know nothing.[vii] Clearly you are capable of impossible things; but since you compel me, I shall answer you. But where shall I begin?

DEL. That is for you to decide.[viii]

2 IL DELFINO, OVERO DEL BACIO   79

PATR. How powerful your magic is! Whoever heard of such a thing, that by watching and observing others one should speak of things he knows he does not know! But tell me, do you believe that every kiss is sweet?
DEL. This I do not know.
PATR. Have you ever been kissed by your father, or by your brother, or another member of your family?
DEL. Yes, I have. But why do you ask me this?
PATR. It is necessary, Mr. Angelo the sorcerer, that I discuss such meaningless questions with you until such time as Love, or one of his spirits, or one of those who obey your enchantments, inspires me to say something of the kiss that is correct and sufficient to satisfy you. Therefore, may it not be burdensome for you to reply to my feeble questions.[ix]
DEL. I shall do exactly that.
PATR. And was the kiss you received from you relatives in any way pleasurable?
DEL. It certainly gave me no pleasure.
PATR. It therefore seems that not every kiss is pleasurable.
DEL. So it seems.
P. And have you ever been kissed on the forehead or cheek?
D. I have.
P. And did you feel any pleasure?
D. I did not.
P. Then what manner of kiss do you consider pleasurable?
D. A kiss on the mouth gives me pleasure.
P. Have you ever been kissed on the mouth by a relative, or a companion, or a friend? For your custom in Venice is to kiss each other when you meet on the road.
D. I have. I do not mean kisses of this kind, but rather those given in acts of love.
P. And if perchance you were with an old or ugly woman, or one with putrid breath, would you take any pleasure then?
D. Let those who wish take pleasure in this way (**107r**), but I do not.
P. And if you received the kisses of a beautiful woman?
D. I would receive them gladly.
P. So you believe that the kiss of every beautiful woman is pleasurable?
D. Yes, I do believe so.
P. Many times I have heard it said by young noblemen that when they are engaged in acts of love with a common woman,[x] however beautiful

she may be they avoid kissing her, almost as if they consider it to be loathsome, rather than sweet.

D. I do not know if I should believe such frivolous things[xi]; but in the case of kisses from a beloved person, what do you say happens?

P. Oh, great providence of Love, how have you led us from such vanities to your marvels? Truly this hermitage is filled with you, and this air is crowded with your sacred spirits. Now, my amorous Mr. Angelo, I am filled with amorous spirits, who will speak sweet words to me with which I may answer your sweet and loving question. Therefore Love, whom I so greatly revere and venerate, awaken your spirits in me, and in this cold hermitage rekindle my heart more than ever before, so that I, as befits your divine flames, might inform this amorous young man of your marvellous and indescribable forces. And you, Mr. Angelo, must pray the same, that Love will be propitious and favourable to us, today and always.

D. And so I pray; but I ask that you answer my question.

P. I believe that indescribable sweetness is found in the kiss of the beloved. And now the spirit[xii] which fills my heart tells me that love alone brings sweetness to the kiss, and without it the kiss is a dead and pleasureless thing.

D. In what manner does this occur?

P. I shall tell you; but do not hinder the spirit that now speaks in me, for he is a good spirit and will not lie to you.

D. I will not, but please continue.

P. Is it not true that the kiss of disfigured women is unpleasant?

D. Certainly it is.

P. That of relatives and friends is not unpleasant, nor does it possess the sweetness of which we speak, which is the property of the loving kiss alone.

D. That is true.

P. Just as there is nothing that burns or heats other than through fire, so no kiss is tempered with sweetness except the loving kiss. Is it not so?

D. Yes, that is true.

P. It is love, therefore, that gives the kiss sweetness, and for this reason the kiss without love it is deprived of sweetness, just as wood without fire does not burn or become hot.

D. You speak the truth.

(**107v**). Pa. Therefore the kiss by its nature does not impart sweetness, for if it by its nature it carried pleasure then the kiss of any person would bring pleasure. This does not happen, for some kisses are unpleasant, and others neither pleasant nor unpleasant.

D. All this is true.

P. Thus love alone brings sweetness to the kiss, for the kiss is only pleasurable between lovers, just as wood only becomes hot if it contains fire.

D. Certainly, the spirit that has entered your heart speaks the truth.

P. Thus the kiss that has been tempered with the sweetness of love yields to lovers the ineffable pleasure they encounter in kissing each other.

D. It alone may do so.

P. But is it the case, Mr. Angelo, that you only take pleasure in the loving kiss upon the mouth?

D. I also take pleasure in the kiss upon the cheek, but not to such an extent.

P. And in kisses elsewhere?

D. Where else? A kiss on the forehead is not a loving kiss, but one of an elder's pure tenderness.

P. Pray, pray to Love that he might show you and reveal all the secrets of his pleasure, for without his grace you will not dare even to gaze upon the deep abyss of his pleasures.

D. And so I pray to him devoutly with my whole heart, that he will make me worthy to consider his marvellous and ineffable pleasures.

P. Now, the amorous spirit within me commands me to tell you that loving kisses are given to the beloved in six places, and in four manners, and no more.

D. And what are these six places?

P. They are the hands, the chest, the neck, the cheeks, the eyes, and the mouth.

D. And the manners?

P. The manners are these: with the joining of lips, with the sucking of the lips, with biting, and with the tongue.[xiii]

D. I thank you, Love, for permitting to receive your secrets; and I pray to you again that through your benevolence you will make me prosperous in them! But you, oh spirit residing in the heart of Patrizio, explain (**108r**) these things to me, each in turn.

P. I shall do so. Of the places, Mr. Angelo, the least pleasant to kiss are the hands, and more pleasant than them is the chest. And what I shall tell you now is a great thing. Although the chest is softer and more delicate than the neck, more pleasure is found in kissing the neck than the chest. There is such sweetness in kissing the neck that while it is not equal to that of the cheeks, which are the chief dwelling place of beauty, it certainly is not far behind them.

D. You speak the truth when you say there is great sweetness in kissing the neck; but I must take your word that it is comparable to that of the cheeks, oh amorous spirit, for I have never tested it.

P. If you do, you will understand that what I tell you is true. The kiss upon the eyes is very sweet, but the kiss upon the mouth surpasses and exceeds the sweetness of all other kisses, even if they are taken all together.

D. Of this, good spirit, I have no doubt.

P. And you must know that this kiss upon the mouth is given in four manners, each sweeter and more pleasant than the next.

D. And what are they?

P. By the joining of lips to lips, the sucking of the beloved's lips, the giving of the tongue, and the receiving it.

D. You speak the truth; and I believe this to be the greatest sweetness that can be felt from the kiss.

P. And yet, Delfino, you have not considered a great difference between the kiss upon the mouth and the other kinds of kiss.

D. Certainly, I have not; but what is it?

P. All kisses, whether on the hands, the chest, the neck, the cheeks, or the eyes, are given; but only that with the mouth is both given and received.

D. I understand.

P. In your opinion, which of the two is sweeter: the kiss given, or the kiss received?

D. As far as I am able to recall at this moment, I feel greater pleasure when the woman kisses me.

P. That is partly true and partly false.

D. How so?

P. Because kisses with the mouth are of three kinds: with the joining of lips, with sucking, and with the tongue.

D. That is true.

P. The first kind, with the lips, gives equal sweetness to both, since neither gives any more than they receive from the other. (**108v**) Therefore, this kiss is less sweet to both lovers than the other two kinds.

D. It is true. But which party takes greater delight in the other two kisses?

P. Undoubtedly the one who loves more strongly.

D. I know this; but if both love each other equally, which of them will experience greater sweetness? The one who gives, or the one who receives?

P. In any kind of kiss the one who receives experiences incomparably greater sweetness than the one who gives.

D. This, spirit, has no semblance of truth.

P. And why not?

D. (It is true that) in the kiss with the tongue the one who receives experiences greater sweetness than the other, who give. Yet it seems to me that in all other kisses the contrary is the case. For in the kiss where the mouth is sucked, the one who sucks, that is who gives, receives greater sweetness than the one who is sucked, who receives. And similarly, the one kissed on the eyes, cheeks, chest, neck or hands receives little or no pleasure, while the one who kisses experiences the utmost pleasure.

P. You argue correctly insofar as the kiss is concerned, Delfino, but I was speaking of another thing.

D. What other thing?

P. Of the cause of the sweetness of the kiss.

D. And what is the cause of this sweetness?

P. The spirit of the beloved, which the lover consumes by kissing.

D. This may well mean something; but I do not understand it, oh gracious spirit.

P. I say that whoever kisses invisibly consumes the spirit of the one kissed, and this is the cause of the great sweetness that is felt in the kiss.

D. In part I understand and in part I do not. It is therefore necessary for you to clarify this matter for me, though it seems that it must be wholly true.

P. It certainly is true, but it is not so easy to explain, for it demands deep contemplation; and so you must pay close attention to what I say.

D. I will pay the closest attention.[xiv]

P. I tell you that two things cause sweetness in the kiss: love, as I said before, and consuming the spirits of the beloved, as I say now. For this reason, kisses given to an unbeloved person give no pleasure, even though their spirit is consumed. (**109r**) And I shall expand on this subject at length, so that you may perfectly understand the mystery of the secret causes of this amorous pleasure that we seek.

D. I ask you this, gentle spirit: that you enlighten me fully, so that I am obliged to praise you.

P. Therefore heed what I say. We must consider two things: the first is how love makes the spirits of the beloved pleasant, and the second is how these spirits are consumed by the lover. And in this regard, I say that love is born in human hearts either from a similarity with another, or from the beauty that another has within themself, or from both of these things conjoined.[xv] Do not be astonished, Delfino, to be told this is true: that woman is most seldom similar to man, and yet she both loves man and is loved by man. For similarity may be external and internal. It is true that external similarity does not cause love at all, but internal similarity is always the cause of love. And such similarity is of two kinds: of the quality of the mind, and of the quality of the body. That of the body exists entirely in the tempering together of the humours and spirits, which compose and give life to the human body. And that of the mind exists in the impressions which, in descending from heaven, two souls from the same ruling planet received within their ethereal body.[xvi] The first similarity, that of the body, is easy to understand, and you will understand this second kind with little effort. You must know that the planets act both upon elemental bodies and upon each another through movement, through light carried by movement, through warmth carried by light, and through the influence of their properties which are carried by warmth. And because warmth and influence depend upon light, the variation of light will result in variation of their actions, caused by the different movements of the planets in the heavens. Depending on the planets' position (**109v**) within the heavens in relation to one another, whether they are closer or more distant, or present one or another of their aspects, they act to a greater or lesser extent upon each other, upon the elements, and upon other bodies. And whenever one of them is more powerful than the others, it is said that he holds dominion. Whoever takes an impression or quality from this dominion takes the name of the ruling planet, be it jovial, or venereal, or any other name. Up to this point I believe you have easily understood.

D. Yes, I certainly understand.

P. Now consider this other point. After it is created by God, the human soul must come to command a terrestrial body. In order that the incorporeal soul may descend to conjoin itself with the corporeal, which is the nature of our elemental body, it invests itself with an ethereal body, by which, almost as an intermediary, it is carried from one extreme up above to another down below. For this reason, some wise men call the ethereal body the vehicle and carriage of the soul.[xvii] And as the soul descends in this body from above the heavens to the earthly element, it takes on light and impressions from each of the planets as it passes through their spheres; but it takes more from those that are in a strong aspect, and more still from the planet which at that time is king over the others. It assumes their qualities in the same way that those who walk in the sun take on a dark colour. And whenever two souls take on qualities and influence from the same ruling planet, or another with strong light, they become similar. The love of which I speak is born from this similarity, or from similarity of temperament, which arises from this in a certain manner, and not from external similarity. And if you sometimes see that a man loves a deformed woman, or on the contrary that a woman loves a loathsome man, it is for this and no other reason.[xviii] And (**110r**) in this way similarity is the cause of love.

D. Now I understand, and I am satisfied concerning this aspect.

P. Furthermore, beauty is the most universal cause of love, for there is no beautiful thing that is not pleasing to all.

D. Do you say this, Patrizio, or is it your spirit that speaks?

P. It seems to me that my spirit is speaking.

D. Do you think it would please him if I were to ask him why it is that beauty is pleasing to all, but not all fall in love?

P. He tells me that I must answer you that there is a most eminent reason for this.

D. And what is it?

P. He says when your soul is formed by its maker, who is full of all the Ideas of things, and before it takes on an ethereal body, it assumes within its substance the causes of all Ideas. In the Intellect they are beautiful creations in the most perfect way possible, and so they remain beautiful in the soul in the most complete manner that its nature permits. Once the celestial body has been formed and clothed in this way, it descends through the heavens and through the elements into the wombs of the mothers of men; and there it gives form to the embryo, receiving the material in the best form, in accordance with the cause of the Idea of the human body that it carries with it. Thus, every soul that descends from the heavens still carries with it the cause of beauty and all its parts. And when we observe them in any body and compare them with the causes our soul carries within itself, they please the soul through their appearance, to a greater or lesser extent according to the degree to which the soul recognises their appearance. For every human soul has such causes of beauty within itself, and each soul, through their recollection, may compare corporeal beauty to its own incorporeal beauty. It is for this-reason (**110v**) that all take pleasure in beauty and its parts. And these are: the proportion of parts of the body, lines, colours, light, shadow, and graces, which are pleasing both together and individually. 'But how do they cause men to fall in love?' you will ask. 'And why not every one?'

D. This is what I seek to know.

P. I say that pleasure, desire, affection, and love are different things. Pleasure is the enjoyment the mind takesin itself, when contemplating beauty that is observed, or another good or perfect thing. But desire is an appetite to possess the thing that causes pleasure; and affection is an inclination to benefit that same thing; and Love is comprised of plea-sure, desire, and affection. Now, I say that in this way all beauty pleases everyone, and after experiencing such pleasure there is no man who does not wish to possess it. Yet this does not mean that every man is inclined to benefit the pleasing and desired thing. That which I called affection becomes love as soon as it is joined with pleasure and desire; but without it, love cannotcome about. Affection certainly is not born of beauty, since all beauty pleases and causes desire of itself, but this does not cause man to fall in love. Rather, love is born of the hidden similarity of which I have told you, for it is seen that when a man happens to meet a person who is neither beautiful not gracious, he is drawn to affection for them by a hidden cause. This cause is nothing other than the similarity we have described, either of the mind or of the body. Now, just as we may find beauty in a person who is not similar to us, so similarity may also be found in a person who is not beautiful. Thus, in the first case pleasure and desire will arise in us, and in the second, affection; but in each these will be separated, for where they are joined (**111r**) together love will arise in us, whenever we find beauty and similarity within the same person.

Truly, then, Love is the coming together of pleasure, desire, and affec-tion. All beauty provokes pleasure and desire of itself in all others, but nevertheless not all fall in love on its account. It is also clear which other beauty it is that makes men fall in love with each other, and why some-times a beautiful man loves a less beautiful woman, or a beautiful woman a less beautiful man.

D. That is so; but it is not yet clear, oh gracious spirit, full of love, why it is that a beautiful woman sometimes loves a loathsome man, or a beautiful man loves a deformed woman.

P. This will be made clear if you consider that one kind of love is brutal and savage, and another is beautiful and worthy of man. The first is entirely inclined towards the depravity of lechery, while the second is entirely inclined towards the enjoyment of conversing and loving beautifully.

D. This is certainly true, but how does it answer my question?

P. It shows that the love between two loathsome people, or one beautiful and one loathsome, is always a brutal and savage love, whose sole purpose is to satisfy the ardent appetites of a depraved soul. But love between a deformed person and a beautiful person, or two who are beautiful, is the better and proper nature of the beautiful manner of love. Thus the first two kinds of love are not always born of similarity; and it is certain they are never born of beauty. They are therefore wholly imperfect kinds of love. But the second two will always be born from similarity and beauty, and thus they are always perfect and complete kinds of love.

D. Now I am contented and satisfied as to my second question. Therefore, oh loving and courteous spirit, return to my first question on the sweetness of kisses. (111v)

P. I shall do so gladly, but you must pay close attention. Beautiful and perfect kinds of love are born from similarity and beauty, and in them by their nature the sweetness of kisses is perfect – which sweetness, as I have said, is scattered within them by love. We may therefore observe in what manner love scatters sweetness within them, and how in this way kisses are so pleasurable. By discussing this, I shall make my principal argument concerning the most noble and beautiful of all kinds of love, in which the sweetness of the kiss is truly perfect.

D. Yes, that is true; but sweetness is not so proper to that kind of love, gentle spirit, that it has no part in the other kind, which is less beautiful.

P. That is true. But this is by accident, not by nature, for the ardent fury that grips man in such love makes what is not sweet appear to be so. However, it is rather imagined and deceitful sweetness, and not the true sweetness we intend to discuss.

D. If that is so, oh spirit full of goodness and virtue, then leave aside speaking of it and instead follow the true and natural sweetness of the kiss.

P. I shall do so. But first, tell me: what is the guide that leads love to human hearts?

D. I do not know that it can be anything other than similarity, of which we have spoken, and beauty.

P. These are the parents and mothers of love, but I ask this: what is the pilot that leads love from similarity and beauty into the human heart?

D. I do not know.

P. The eyes, which are none other than a gateway through which love passes, oh men, from similar beauty into your soul.

D. And how does it pass through them, oh amorous spirit?

P. It does so because the rays of the eyes (**112r**) carry both the luminescence of similar beauty and the spirits of the heart.[xx] When these rays are fixed upon your eyes, they cast themselves into your heart, and the spirits impress within it an image of the beauty from which they come and kindle it with their flames. These are the true darts, arrows, and sparks by which Love pierces and enflames the hearts of others and within them makes such sweet wounds and such ardent flames, so that however much sweetness is subsequently consumed they are never healed or reduced. Amorous Delfino, have you ever burned with love of this kind?

D. Yes, gentle spirit, and indeed I am at this very moment. But tell me at greater length of this entry of the rays and spirits of others into our hearts.

P. I shall do so willingly. The first thing you must know is that universally within all eyes is found both a great diversity of colours, or of clarity, and a great multitude of spirits and rays. But none has so many spirits and rays, and thus shines as brightly, as that which you commonly call the glad eye, and for this reason it makes others fall in love more than any other. And the glad eye is of two colours and no more: black and blue, which the common people call white. Those in between these colours are not glad eyes, or they are only to the degree that they have one or the other of the aforesaid colours. Of these, it is doubtless black that makes the most beautiful sight, contrasting with the white flesh of the eye, and it is commonly judged the most beautiful. But in truth, it is blue that makes others fall in love more swiftly. This is for no other reason than the pairing of spirits and rays, which are the true arrows of love, and the invisible spark with which he sets alight the souls of others.

D. This, (**112v**) gentle spirit, I believe to be true. But in order that I am better prepared, you must demonstrate it to me more clearly.

P. I will not tire of satisfying your questions all day, so long as you listen to me.

D. And I will not tire of listening to you in a hundred years, oh gentle and noble spirit. Nor could you give me any sweeter or more pleasant nourishment than you give me now, for which I consider myself eternally beholden to you.

P. Therefore listen to me attentively. All things enacted by Mother Nature have as their father the Sun, and each retains its paternal qualities according to their power. Some retain its light, others its colour, which is illumination clothed in material, and others still retain both light and colour. Such are precious stones and the eyes of animals, which more than any other thing have colour and light. And since each body that has light spreads the rays of its light, which carry within themselves illumination in order to brighten the dark air around them, the aforementioned stones, and the eyes of animals and of man, have both light and rays.[xxiii] Of this, Delfino, you must harbour no doubt,[xiv] for we may observe that nocturnal birds and animals have eyes that are clear and bright at night; and while you may not see so clearly with your own eyes, it is nevertheless true that they are luminous. If another places their finger over the corner of your eye nearest the nose, you will see there a little circle full of illumination. This is certain proof of the light of your eyes, which in you men as in the aforesaid animals emits rays from itself. This is plainly demonstrated by observation. The animals I have mentioned see clearly at night, which they certainly could not do if the rays of their eyes did not illuminate the dark air around them; and you would not see the brightness of their eyes if it (**113r**) were not transported to your own eyes by their rays. There is no stronger proof of this than that if the aforesaid animals fix their eyes upon the ground, or on any other thing that is firm and distinct, a small luminous circle is formed opposite their eyes, corresponding with the pupil. This cannot be caused by anything other than the rays of their eyes, which carry the light of their eyes to the point at which they finish. The same is true of human eyes: for when Marius was imprisoned in a dark place, he shocked the man who had been sent by Sulla to kill him with the light of his eyes.[xxiv] And when Tiberius was awakened at night in a dark place, he was able to see all that was there for a short while[xxv]; this can only have happened because the rays of his eyes carried illumination with them for that time. And Augustus had such strong visual rays, and so full of light, that if he stared into the eyes of another that man would be forced to look elsewhere, as if blinded.[xxvi] This can only be because the excessive illumination of his rays dispersed those of the other, and forced him to flee. Because of these many and strong proofs, oh Delfino, I contend that you believe human eyes have light within themselves, and from themselves send out luminous rays.

D. So I believe, without doubt.

P. Therefore I shall now speak of spirits, which are the second quality of eyes that cause others to fall in love, beginning from here. The spirit, understood in a human sense, is nothing other than a most subtle vapour of the blood, which is generated in the heart by its natural heat. This spirit carries the heat of the heart through the veins, which physicians call arteries, to all of the particles of the living body, even the very smallest, which keep it hot and alive. The spirit is the true enactor of the heat and life of others; and since everything that is hot and (113v) subtle by its nature rises upwards, a large part of the spirit, which is so, rises from the body to the head and the brain, and is further purified by its temperature. Here, the spirit becomes an instrument not of life but of powerful knowledge of the soul and bodily movements. It is naturally sent through appropriate vessels to the instruments of sense and will, and to the nerves of motion, by which man moves and senses. Here, two vessels in the form of veins pass from the ventricles of the brain and carry the spirit that has been purified there to the eyes. Because these veins are very broad, they carry a great abundance of the spirit to the eyes; and since the spirit is itself clear, when its clarity mixes with the natural clarity of the eyes, it makes this part of animals and men bright, much more so than all the other parts.

D. It can well be seen, oh gentle spirit, that the eyes are the clearest of all parts. But how do you prove that the spirit augments their clarity?

P. There is clear proof of this, for all hot and subtle bodies possess clarity. And moreover, there is a second proof: for it is evident that a living man's eye is much clearer than that of a dead man. The sole cause is that the living man has more spirit than the dead man. This is itself confirmed by another example, for when the pupil of the eye is large, it shines more brightly than when it is small on account of some exertion; and this is because when the spirits of the head are consumed in exertion, they do not flow to the eye so copiously.

D. Of this I am satisfied, gracious spirit.

P. When the spirit reaches the extremities of the body, it is pushed by the beating of the heart and the movements of the limbs through little visible and hidden openings in the skin, which you men call pores, by which it exits and is dispersed. And the same occurs through openings in the eyes, which are identical in that place to the rest of your body. When the spirit exits through these openings in the eyes, (114r) which it does readily as through those of the body, it joins and unites with the rays of the eyes, and travels with them until its force is opposed by external forces, and it maintains its state. But as soon as the spirit is extinguished by opposing forces, the ray is left without it.

D. This follows, good and wise spirit; but how do you prove the union between spirit and ray? I find it very difficult to comprehend.

P. I will demonstrate it by two proofs. The first is seen in a woman at the time of her bleeding, who upon looking into a mirror observes that it is stained with droplets of blood. This is nothing other than the spirit, which, damp with blood, is carried by the ray to the surface of the mirror, and on account of its cold temperature turns into droplets.[xxvii]

D. If this is true, it is a very great proof.

P. You may observe it at your leisure. I have heard several times from a philosophical spirit, who is my friend, that he demonstrated it to Aristotle, who then wrote about it in his books. But the other proof is that if a man looks for any length of time into the eyes of another who is unwell, he himself will become similarly unwell[xxviii]; and this, I assure you, is what happened to Petrarch when he looked into the right eye of his Laura. I know that he wrote of this in his amorous passions, and you young lovers would do well to heed it.

D. Yes, he did so in that sonnet: *Qual ventura mi fu quando dall'uno* (*What chance befell me when, from one*).[xxix]

P. And this is not spell or enchantment, but rather natural force. Nature does not enact its effects without a means to do so; and between her eye and his, I know that the means was the passing of the ray and the spirit of which I speak, and that it was the spirit that carried that illness into the eye of Petrarch. But now we have reached the course through which love passes into your soul, and it is necessary that you pay the closest attention, Delfino.

D. I will pay the closest attention.

P. When the spirit exits the eye together with a luminous ray, it seeks the eye of another. If one of these eyes is much clearer than the other, it will overcome and blind it, in the same way that Augustus blinded the eyes of others. When it blinds the other eye, it enlarges its pores, and the spirit, augmented by the force of the (**114v**) gaze, penetrates within. Finding that the spirits within are not enemies, but rather brothers born under the same dominium, it willingly mixes with them; and in their company, for they are just as subtle, it proceeds to seek the heart where the others were born, a place naturally dear to them and their keeper. Once the foreign spirit has been brought by the native spirit to the heart, and has subtly penetrated its substance, it inflames the heart more than ever before, and on account of the similarity it has acquired by its intimacy with the native spirits, it willingly makes its home there, as if it had returned to its proper place. This new guest is sweet and comes from a similar and not hateful heart; so, when the heart discovers it, it welcomes and retains it gladly. This philosophy, Delfino, is proper to enamoured intellects. Moreover, since when it entered through the eyes the foreign spirit carried with it the image of beauty from which it derives, it now shapes the spirits of the heart in which it dwells according to that same beauty. The rational soul sees and recognises in the spirits a beauty that is very similar to the cause it has within it of the beauty of the human body, and it compares that beauty to the cause. In this comparison, it invariably happens that the contemplative soul deceives itself on account of that marvellous beauty and the loveliness of that similarity, and adds the perfection of its cause to the defects of that beauty. From this error is born a further error common to lovers, who always consider the beauty of the beloved to be greater than it truly is.[xxx] This, amorous Delfino, is how love enters into your hearts; and the flames and sweetness felt in the heart of the enamoured man are caused by the heat and similarity of the foreign spirits that have entered there. In such a way love makes the spirits of the beloved sweet and gentle, since through them (**115r**) he has sweetened the spirits of the lover and made them similar to those of the beloved.

D. You have revealed beautiful and marvellous secrets to me, most amorous spirit. But tell me, I ask you, virtuous spirit: how does the gaze of the luminous and beautiful eyes of the woman have the force to make her spirits pass into the hearts of others and enflame them with love? And do those of the man, although they are luminous, not have the same force to make their spirits pass into the heart of the woman, and make her likewise fall in love?

P. I have already told you, Delfino, that if the spirit is not very clear and copious, so that by blinding another's eye it opens its pores and enters therein, then it does not have the power to kindle the flame of love in any heart. Hence it happens only rarely, if ever, that anyone falls in love except by means of clear and bright eyes. For this reason, if a woman happens upon a young man's eyes that are luminous and full of spirit, which are fixed upon her own, mutual flames of love will be kindled in both her and him. But if the eyes of the young man are not very luminous, and thus not capable of kindling love in her, she will nevertheless retain amorous affection for him on account of the similarity between them. This happens even if she is not at all enflamed because she has not received that dart from him. Here, Delfino, I assure you that no woman ever makes another fall in love with her unless she herself is smitten with love, or at least with affection for the beloved. For which reason you must always be more willing to love, since you can be certain the feeling will either be requited, or only a little less than mutual.

D. This is such good news, gentle spirit, that if only lovers heard it, they would shower you with thanks. And I for my part will tell it to all who I meet (**115v**), for I am eternally indebted to you.

P. Please do so, Delfino; but let us continue. When the soul is imprinted with the beauty of another, it conserves that image safely and in its entirety for a long time. But since spirits are subtle substances, and gradually dispersed by the continued labour of the heart, when they are deprived of the sweetness of the heat of others and the sweetness of company they continuously desire to renew themselves and receive new brothers. From here is born the ardent desire to see again the eyes of the beloved, in which I know that Petrarch felt such sweetness that he considered all the other pleasures experienced by lovers to be nothing. Thus, lovers desire to see the beloved person again, and especially their eyes, in order to renew their flames and the sweetness the heart derives from the company of its guest. But what, you will ask, causes the desire to touch the beloved? And the sweetness of the kiss? That, Delfino, was your first question.

D. So it was, gentle spirit; now, come to it at last.

P. I answer you that there is no cause other than that renewal of the ardour and joy of the heart, which happens in this way. The heart by its nature contracts and expands, and when it expands it draws air to itself from the lungs, which in turn draw it from the nose and mouth; and it also draws in air through the whole of the skin by those small openings named pores, which lead to insensible arteries, which I termed the vessels and channels of the spirits. When the heart contracts, it instead empties itself of spirits and air, and the spirits are propelled through the arteries to their mouths and arrive at the skin (**116r**), where they exit the body through the said openings. The heart does this continuously while it is alive, in order to renew and refresh its spirits and its heat, which is necessary to keep it alive.[xxxii] Now, Delfino, heed what I say. Since the enamoured heart is a heart, it seeks to renew its spirits; but since it is an enamoured heart, it seeks renewal of its joy, which is lessened and found wanting due to the dispersal of those spirits. It may be renewed by brothers of those first spirits, which may come either by seeing the eyes of the beloved again or, more abundantly, by touching the beloved person. For when the beloved is touched, the enamoured heart attempts to draw in air through natural motion by means of the arteries, but instead it draws in the spirits of the beloved. Having sent them out of his heart by the same means, he draws them in instead of the air and sweetly restores himself; and so he senses renewed flames and sweetness. I shall offer two certain arguments to demonstrate that this is true.[xxxiii] The first is this: the more parts of his body the lover uses to touch the beloved, the greater ardour and joy he feels; and the fewer, the less ardour and joy. And this stands to reason, for in the first instance he draws in the spirits of the beloved through a greater number of arteries, and in the second through fewer arteries, and receives fewer spirits. The second proof is that if for any reason the body of the beloved is cold when the lover touches it, he receives little or no sweetness or fire. This is because the cold by its nature causes the pores to contract, so that the spirits of the beloved may not pass through them, and consequently the pores of the beloved may not draw them in. And, if you wish, a third proof is that the lover derives considerably more sweetness by clasping the beloved to himself than he does by simply touching the beloved. This is because (**116v**) that clasping forces both hearts to struggle somewhat, and hence both are compelled to emit and draw in the spirits of the other with greater force and more abundantly; for which reason, by emitting them more abundantly and more copiously drawing in those of the other, they more copiously feel both sweetness and ardour. But now I come to the kiss. The kiss is sweet to the beloved for this reason alone: he draws to himself and consumes the spirits of the beloved, whether he kisses the hand, chest, neck, cheek, eyes or mouth. For the same reason the sucking kiss is sweeter than the joining of lips, for not only does it gather those spirits that are emitted by the beloved heart, but it draws in others by force, and all are consumed. The sucking kiss upon the mouth is furthermore sweeter than elsewhere, for the broader aperture allows for more spirits to be drawn in than through the small openings in the skin. Even sweeter than this sucking kiss is the kiss with the tongue, for it not only draws in the same abundance of spirits, but a far greater number, since it draws in those of the tongue, which is a spongy body and always full, and even tastes of the inner humour of the beloved body. This humour contains heat and spirits mixed together, which when they are conjoined and drawn from the beloved heart cause the beating, enfeeblement and exhaustion within it that makes the body of the other become suddenly numb, immobile and insensible.

D. Now I am satisfied, and entirely contented; and now, thanks to you, courteous spirit, I understand these high marvels and sweet secrets. But tell me one final thing, amorous spirit: what of that biting kiss, and kisses upon the other parts you have mentioned?

P. The biting kiss does not allow the lover (**117r**) to draw to himself more spirits than the sucking kiss; but since he burns for that person, and in his heart is offended by her, he is compelled by a sudden desire for revenge on she who possesses him, and he takes up those arms that are most ready. But realising that he has life through her, he swiftly repents and turns that revenge to sweet nourishing of his flames. Hands are kissed as they are ministers of the thoughts of the beloved heart. The chest is kissed as their abode. But for the present, Delfino, Love does not wish that I reveal to you why the kissing of the neck brings such sweetness. Pray to him devoutly that, at least in the future, he might deign to reveal this secret to you, and to explain another concerning the same kiss; which is that much greater sweetness is derived from kissing the left part of the neck than the right.[xxxvi] But the cheek is kissed as the true abode of the beauty of the face, because it is the seat of the colours that produce it and the vivacity of the eyes. The eyes are kissed as the first and most potent cause of the flames and joys of others. Finally, the mouth is kissed because it is the opening of the soul and the heart, and the broadest channel for the spirits of the beloved, and more copious and abundant than any other thing. And the kiss on the chest is sweeter than that upon the hands, because the spirits consumed there are newer and closer to the heart that produces them. The sweetness caused by kissing the cheeks is in part the opinion of the lover, who believes he is consuming the beloved beauty wholly and in its entirety. You have already heard of the cause of the kiss on the mouth and its sweetness. It stands to reason that the kiss on the eyes increases the sweetness of the other parts, except the mouth, for the lover, wounded by their sweet and pleasurable arrows, in kissing them comforts his wounds and drinks in new sweetness with new spirits.[xxxvii] But Love does not wish for me to explain to you the kiss upon the neck until such time as you have offered a worthy sacrifice to him.[xxxviii]

D. And what sacrifice is fitting to him, oh good and amorous spirit? But Patrizi, he does not reply.

P. He will certainly speak no more, for he has answered your questions.

D. Oh Love, most powerful God, I thank you with all my soul, for today you have deigned to reveal to me so many of your marvellous secrets, high secrets which have never before been made apparent to any man. (117v) I sacrifice this soul and this heart to you, if they are worthy of your divinity; and if they are not, I devoutly pray that you reveal to me what burnt offerings might please you, so that I may demonstrate my gratitude for the many benefits received from you, today and always. This I ask you, so that if I am lacking in my debt, I shall not provoke your anger against me, to whom you are always propitious and favourable (Fig. 2.1).

I saw Love, who in the pale, beautiful chest
        Of my idol went tending those dear, sweet spirits,
        And with sweet, greedy kisses
        Filled himself with their sweetness.
The soul, overcome by envy,
        Hurried there, and hungering for those clear celestial spirits,
        He made off, imbibing them;
        And never shall he be sated.
Love, who was seen deprived of such sweet life,
        With fiery brand burned his wings,
        And he can return to me no more.
My Idol, so that I may return to you alive,
        Let me, I pray, with my weak lips
        Gather the soul within your beautiful chest.[xxxix]

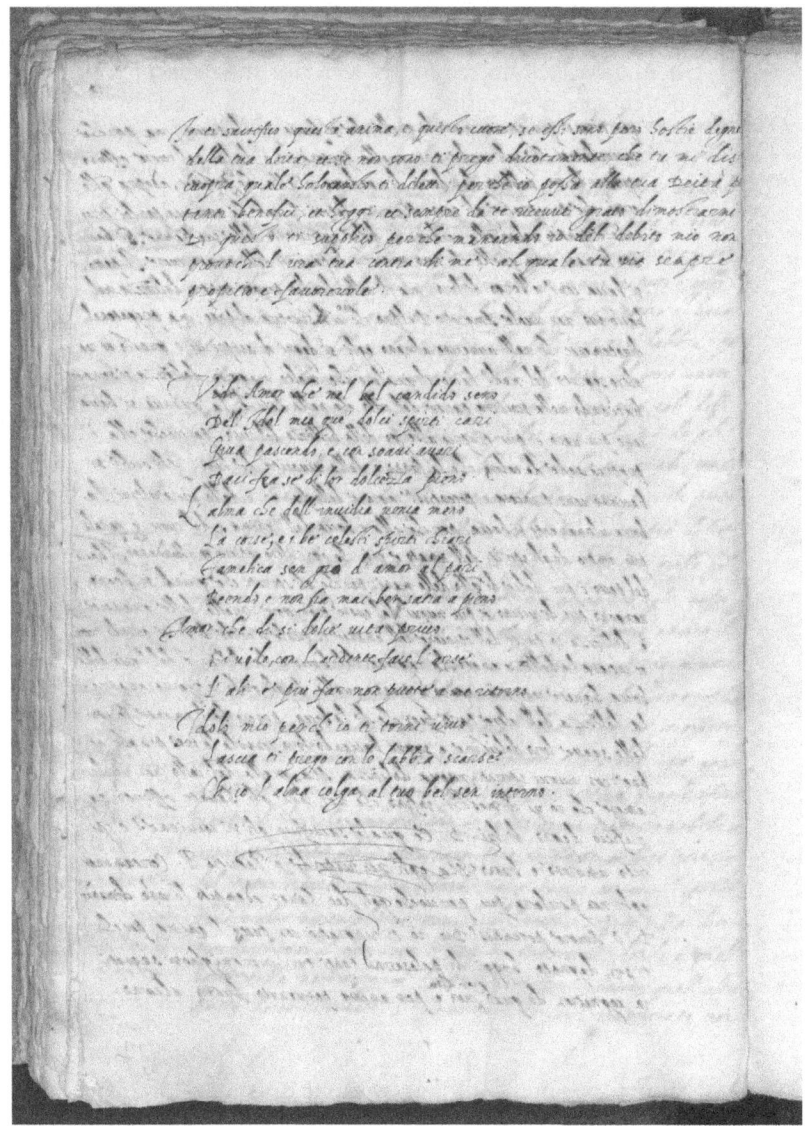

Fig. 2.1 Final folio of the manuscript: MS Q 119 sup., fol. 117v, Milan, Biblioteca Ambrosiana

COMMENTARY NOTES

i. On Angelo Delfino see footnote **51** of the introductory essay. The choice of interlocutor may be motivated by Patrizi's connections with the Venetian nobility, as well as the correspondence between the family name and the dolphin (which appears in its coat of arms): an animal sacred to Venus that therefore echoes the amorous subject matter of the dialogue.

ii. The dialogue commences *in medias res* and the location and precise occasion of the meeting between Delfino and Patrizi are not specified. Delfino opens the dialogue and it may be hypothesised that within its fiction the young man has called upon Patrizi in his house. Given the esoteric tone the dialogue swiftly assumes, it is plausible to imagine the scene taking place in a room within a private dwelling, a quiet and secluded space. Patrizi identifies himself as a hermit shortly afterwards, and it is reasonable to assume his dwelling lies outside of the city.

iii. The subject of the *kiss* is not entirely novel within treatises on love. The philosophical tradition had already approached the kiss from a mystical and metaphysical perspective, beginning from the kabbalistic theme of the *binsica* (or the death of the kiss). Giovanni Pico della Mirandola explores this theme within a discussion of the philosophy of love in his *Commentary on a canzone of Girolamo Benivieni* (1486). The kiss is also presented through a specifically human lens in the fourth book of the *Courtier*, where Baldassare Castiglione interprets the phenomenon in broadly ethical terms, albeit through a not entirely coherent analysis. It is likely that Patrizi's underlining of the originality of the subject is largely a polemical strategy in relation to these earlier and widely disseminated works. He is indeed the first to approach the question through an almost entirely physiological paradigm, as emerges in the course of the dialogue; see the introductory essay (**pp. 26–27**). After the *Delfino*, the question of the kiss is also confronted—though without reaching Patrizi's naturalistic heights—in Flaminio Nobili's *Treatise on Human Love* (*Trattato dell'Amore Humano*, 1567) and Annibale Romei's *Discourses* (*Discorsi*, 1586) (specifically the discourse on human love). Patrizi himself appears as a principal interlocutor in the

latter work, albeit not in the discourse on human love but
another dedicated to beauty.

iv. The figure of the wise hermit (the so-called *romito*) had
become topical in the wake of Pietro Bembo's *Asolani*. In this
widely read dialogue, which sets in motion the gradual transformation of the genre of the love treatise into a literary *trend*
(see the introductory essay, **pp. 26–28**), Bembo reveals the
profound and sacred secrets of love through the figure of the
wise hermit ('at one of its corners, I became aware, a hut was
built, and not far off there slowly moved among the trees a
solitary figure, a bearded, white-haired man clothed in a material like the bark of the young oaks surrounding him. He had
not perceived me; and deep in thought, it seemed, he sometimes stopped in his perambulation and after a little began
pacing slowly again. He had done this many times when it
struck me he must be that holy man who I had heard was
living as a *hermit* in this neighbourhood, to which he had
come in order that he might, by studying sacred books, the
better to pursue his lofty contemplations' (Pietro Bembo, *Gli
Asolani*, (Bloomington: Indiana University Press, 1954): 168–
169, (III-11, 169, my italics)); 'così dall'uno de' canti mi
venne una capannuccia veduta, et poco dallei discosto tra gli
alberi un huom tutto solo lentamente passeggiare, canutissimo
et barbuto et vestito di panno simile alle corteccie de' quer-
ciuoli, tra' quali egli era. Non s'era costui aveduto di me, il
quale in profondo pensiero essendo, sì come a me parea di
vedere, tale volta nello spatiare si fermava et, stato ched egli
era così un poco, a passeggiare lento lento si ritornava; et così
più volte fatto havea, quando io mi pensai che questi potesse
essere quel santo huomo, che io havea udito dire che a guisa
di *romito* si stava in questo dintorno, venutovi per meglio
potere, nello studio delle sante lettere dimorando, pensare
alle alte cose' (Bembo, *Gli Asolani*, (III-11), 329–330). The
passage contains various echoes of the holy solitude of the
figure of Diotima in the *Symposium* (201d), where the most
sacred and profound amorous secrets are similarly revealed by
an individual in direct contact with the divine and isolated
from human company. Patrizi seems here to present himself
as a hermit precisely in reference to this tradition, adopting a

perspective that is a times parodic. Indeed, how can an individual removed from human company understand a subject like love, which, with all due respect to Bembo's hermit and Diotima, has inevitable and decidedly worldly implications? One detail worthy of our attention—apparently of secondary importance, but this is potentially misleading—is the implication of Patrizi's self-identification as a hermit, but not an *old* hermit. We might customarily associate the wisdom of the hermit with the wisdom of advanced age, as in the *Asolani*; however, here this is not the case. Patrizi employs the precisely same term, *romito*, to identify himself in another composed around the same time as the *Delfino*, his *Dialogues on History* (1560). Here, he writes that upon returning to his native island of Cres following his university studies in Padua, 'having been assailed by melancholy, he was taken by the quartan fever; and after eleven months of healing, in order to consume the remains of that malign humour, he had sought (not understanding medicine) a remedy that was inconvenient to him. This was withdrawing to a life of solitude, in which I lived as a *romito* (hermit) for over a year' (Francesco Patrizi, *Della Historia. Diece dialoghi di M. Francesco Patritio ne'quali si ragiona di tutte le cose appartenenti all'historia, e allo scriverla, e all'osservarla* (Venice: A. Arrivabene, 1560): 54v, my italics). Beyond the surprising admission concerning his knowledge of medicine, which seems improbable given his studies in Padua, what is significant here is that around 1555, and therefore at the age of about 26 years old, the author describes himself as a hermit—and certainly not an old one. This correspondence between *On History* and the *Delfino* points towards a juvenile dating of the latter work (see Bolzoni, *A proposito di una recente edizione*, 148–149). If, on the contrary, we twist the text to read Patrizi's self-identification in the *Delfino* as that of an *old* hermit (as Danilo Aguzzi Barbagli does in the introduction to his *Lettere ed opuscoli inediti*, XXIII), the consequent dating of the work to his later years introduces a whole series of chronological contradictions (see the *Critical note*).

v. This claim about Patrizi is reaffirmed in the later dialogue on *The Philosophy of Love*, where the poet Tarquinia Molza, the protagonist of the work, directly tells the philosopher that 'I have known about this for a long time – that all the Platonists both say and want to be in love in their entire lives. Similarly, you, too, since you say you are a Platonist, are also consequently in love' (Patrizi, *The Philosophy of Love*, 111). An earlier line with similar implications is voiced by Giulio Carrato, who admits: 'We know that Patrizi is so truthful and has such refined judgment – especially in matters of love and beauty' (Patrizi, *The Philosophy of Love*, 34). The strong and evidently widespread connection between certain expressions of Platonism and reflections on love and beauty doubtless traces its origin to Ficino. In the sixteenth century, this connection was increasingly radicalised, as demonstrated by Patrizi, who presented himself as closely involved in questions of beauty and love throughout his intellectual career. He nevertheless invariably strives to differentiate his own reflections from more frivolous discussions of this cultural touchstone, which was increasingly fashionable among non-experts; see the introductory essay (**pp. 26–27**) and Ghezzani, *Il Platonico Innamorato*, especially XIX–XXXIII.

vi. Recourse to the sensible experience of the 'proof', along with rational demonstration and references to authoritative sources, is characteristic of Patrizi's inquiry. In the opening of his philosophical masterpiece, the *New Philosophy of the Universe* (*Nova de universis philosophia*), he writes 'Franciscus Patricius, Novam, Veram, Integram, de universis conditurus Philosophiam, sequentia, uti verissima, pronunciare est ausus. Pronunciata, *ordine* persecutus, *Divinis oraculis, Geometricis necessitatibus, Philosophicis rationibus, clarissimisque experimentis comprobavit*' (Francesco Patrizi, *Nova de universis philosophia, in qua aristotelica methodo non per motum sed per lucem, et lumina, ad primam causam ascenditur. Deinde propria Patricii methodo, tota in contemplationem venit Divinitas. Postremo methodo Platonica, rerum universitas, a conditore Deo deducitur* (Ferrara: B. Mammarelli, 1591), 1r, my italics). In short, he guarantees the accuracy of his philosophical system through not only continuity with the sources of his knowledge, but also rational evidence, marked by the rigour of order, and specifically through consistency with sensible experience. In the *Delfino*, theoretical results are almost always corroborated by evidence taken from sensible experience. In this regard, Patrizi's education at the University of Padua may have played a more than negligible role, despite his reluctance to admit so openly. For all his negative judgement of his tutors in logic and philosophy, he nevertheless admits an appreciation for the methodological approach of the physicians Bassiano Lando and Giovanni Battista da Monte (see the introductory essay, **pp. 24–25**).

vii. During the Renaissance (and beyond), the theme of magic was closely connected to that of love. Here too the founding paradigm is to be found in Ficino. In *On the Nature of Love*, he develops the passage in the *Symposium* where the god Love is defined among other things as a magician ('[Love] is a genius at magic and an expert in the use of words and herbs' (Plato, *Symposium*, 53)). Ficino asks 'But why is Love called a magician? It is because the whole power of magic consists of love. The work of magic is to attract one thing to another through natural likeness. The parts of this cosmos, like the limbs of an animal, all dependent on a single Author, are joined together through a natural communion. [...] Thus the operations of magic are the operations of nature, and art is its handmaiden. For when art perceives that in some place there is not total harmony among the different natures, she compensates for this, at the right times' (M. Ficino, *On the Nature of Love*, (VI-10), 105–106) ('Ma perché si chiama l'Amore mago? Perché tutta la forza della magica consiste nello amore: l'opera della magica è uno certo tiramento dell'una cosa dall'altra per similitudine di natura. Le parti di questo mondo, come membri d'uno animale dependendo tutte da uno Auctore, si connectono insieme per comunione di natura [...]. Adunque l'opere della magica sono opere della natura, e l'arte è ministra; perché l'arte, quando s'avede che in qualche parte non è intera convenientia tra le nature, supplisce a questo in tempi debiti' (*El libro dell'amore*, (VI-10, 144–145)). In other words, from the moment a connection—of precisely a *passionate* nature— is established in the divine plan between reality, physics, and metaphysics, magic can be understood as the continuation and strengthening of providential action through the control of this connection. Ficino understands the magician as a philosopher who has attained knowledge of the universal architecture and the analogical forces that govern it, the forces of amorous nature, and who is thus capable of actively controlling those laws. Nevertheless, in this case the author appears to resort to the theme of the amorous enchantment as a rhetorical and narrative device, rather than for its theoretical value. Ficino was among the first to assess the capability of magical enchantments to grant the summoner and/or those around him access to profound and high knowledge (see, for example, Ficino, *Three Books on Life*, (III-21), 354–363). For a general overview of the phenomenon of magic in the early modern period, along with further bibliography, see in particular Walker, *Spiritual and Demonic Magic*; Frances A. Yates, *Giordano Bruno and the Hermetic Tradition* (Chicago: University of Chicago Press, 1964): 1–189; Couliano, *Eros and Magic in the Renaissance*; E. Garin, *Ermetismo del Rinascimento* (Pisa: Edizioni della Normale, 2006); Germana Ernst and Guido Giglioni (edited by), *I vincoli della natura. Magia e stregoneria nel Rinascimento* (Rome: Carocci, 2012); Dario Gurashi, *In deifico speculo. Agrippa's humanism* (Paderborn: Brill-Fink, 2021).

viii. This line concludes the introductory section of the text. The following section is dedicated to defining the subject of the dialogue, the amorous kiss, and is characterised by the so-called Socratic method of *maieutics*. Through an intense sequence of questions posed by Patrizi, Delfino comes ever closer to the truth. To a certain extent, this section mirrors the passage of the *Symposium* (201d-209e) in which the young Socrates (whose equivalent here is Delfino) is instructed in the first part of amorous mysteries by the priestess Diotima (Patrizi), again through the Socratic method.

ix. Unlike Diotima, in this section of the text the character of Patrizi lacks any knowledge of the higher amorous truths, and his insights are therefore more straightforward. He continues in the expectation that some amorous spirit—which is to say some *demon*, an intermediate being between human beings and more transcendent realities—will reveal deeper knowledge to him. Despite a reluctance in many Renaissance magical treatises to discuss them directly, demons could be summoned by the magician, and once *captured* could reveal their knowledge to him. On this subject, see for instance Maude Vanhaelen, 'Cosmic Harmony, Demons, and the Mnemonic Power of Music in Renaissance Florence. The Case of Marsilio Ficino' in *Sing Aloud Harmonious Spheres. Renaissance Conceptions of Cosmic Harmony*, edited by Jacomien Prins and Maude Vanhaelen (New York: Routledge, 2017).

x. Or rather with a prostitute.

xi. Delfino is clearly sceptical as to the status of the pleasure derived from a prostitute's kisses. He expresses his doubts in similar fashion at various other points during the dialogue. This most likely points towards a strategy adopted by the author not only to make the text more dynamic, but also to better depict the character of his young interlocutor.

xii. From here on, Patrizi functions as an intermediary for the spirit (his reluctance to refer to it as a demon should be noted), who reveals the profound secrets of the kiss to Delfino. This passage marks a departure from the questions that precede it, which the character of Patrizi considers himself capable of answering without special knowledge, and a transition to more complex matters. The close dialogue between Patrizi and Delfino is increasingly replaced by a single voice, that of Patrizi possessed by the spirit, which delivers long monologues. The section of the *Symposium* dedicated to the young Socrates and Diotima follows a similar pattern: the priestess delivers a monologue on the higher mysteries of Love, while Socrates remains silent (209e–212a).

xiii. On this taxonomy of kisses see the table in the introductory essay (**p. 30**). In addition to the identification of the kiss on the mouth as the most pleasurable, the list of parts of the body is similar to one that appears in a widely disseminated sixteenth-century work: Johannes Secundus, *Basia* in Id., *The Love Poems* (London: G. Routledge, 1930): 72. See also Vuilleumier Laurens, 'Les Basia de Jean Second et la tradition philosophique de Marsile Ficin à Francesco Patrizi'.

xiv. Here, the section dedicated to defining the subject of the dialogue comes to an end. The text will now turn to more demanding content, for in order to explain the pleasure

deriving from various kinds of kiss it is necessary to introduce the cornerstones of the philosophy and physiology of love.
These will be presented in the following order: love as deriving
from beauty and the astrological similarity of lovers; the theory
of the *spiritus* and ocular rays; the necessity of renewing the
spiritus through touch.

xv. Beauty and similarity are here presented as distinct concepts.
In Platonic thought, and for Ficino specifically, similarity was
considered a particular kind of beauty; see the introductory
essay (**pp. 30–31**).

xvi. The following discussion (continuing to D **62–64**) of the ethereal body, astral similarity and anamnesis is derived from Ficino
(*On the Nature of Love*, VI-4, VI-6), 117–119, 122–125); see
the introductory essay (**pp. 8–14, 31–32**).

xvii. The primary source of this image is the myth of the chariot of
the soul as narrated in the *Phaedrus* (246a).

xviii. This final reiteration of the distinction between beauty and
similarity is obviously absent in Ficino.

xix. The distinctions are invariably based on the conceptual distinction between beauty and similarity.

xx. Ficino (*On the Nature of Love*, (VII-4–10), 189–206) is the
source of the following discussion (continuing to D **73–74**)
of falling in love through transmission of the *spiritus* via ocular
rays and the compulsion, experienced by the lover, to renew
one's own *spiritus* with that of the beloved. Here, Ficino's
entirely negative opinion of this process, which he conceives
as the transmission of a disease, is obviously overturned; see
the introductory essay (**pp. 13–24, 31–41**).

xxi. The following discussion presents different kinds of eyes with
reference to the theory of the 'glad eye'. It resumes and
develops a brief passage of Ficino, who in reality is concerned
with the different types of humoral complexion. Ficino states
that the masculine complexion is more capable of making
others fall in love than its feminine counterpart. Having blue
eyes is one of the characteristics that make certain men more
adept in this regard (*On the Nature of Love*, (VII-9), 147:
'Someone may ask, "By what kinds of people in particular, and
in what way, are lovers ensnared? And how are they set free?"
Men are easily caught by women, and even more easily by

women who display some masculine characteristics. Still more easily do men catch men, for they bear a closer resemblance to them than do women, and their blood and spirit are clearer, warmer and finer; and this is how Cupid's nets close in. The men who are quickest at putting the evil eye on men and women are those who are sanguine to the highest degree and choleric to the lowest degree, and who have large, blue and shining eyes. This is especially true if they live chaste lives, for through the practice of coitus their clear spirits disperse and their bodies grow dark'; (*El libro dell amore*, (VII-9), 203: 'Dimanderà forse alcuno da quali persone maxime e in che modo s'allacciano gli amanti, e in che modo si sciolgono. Le femmine pigliano e maschi facilmente, e quelle femmine più facilmente che mostrano qualche masculina effigie; e maschi ancora più facilmente pigliano gli huomini, essendo a·lloro più simili che le femmine e avendo el sangue e lo spirito più lucido, più caldo e più sottile, nella qual cosa s'appiccano le reti di Cupidine. E del numero de' maschi più velocemente fanno mal d'occhio a' maschi o alle femmine quegli, e quali nel maggior grado sono sanguigni e nel minore collerici, e hanno gli occhi grandi, azzurri e splendidi, spetialmente se casti vivono; imperò che per l'uso del coito, risolvendosi e chiari spiriti, el corpo fusco diventa'). Since Ficino excludes carnality, which he considers a disease, the claim that men are more capable of provoking erotic desire in other men does not appear problematic from the perspective of religious orthodoxy. Given that Patrizi legitimises the carnality of love at various points in his discussion, he likely considered it inconvenient to resume Ficino's reflection on the greater erotic power of the masculine complexion, and he instead dwells solely on the eyes. For similar reasons, and taking the matter further, he speaks exclusively of heterosexual couples. The theory of the glad eye is also present in Castiglione and Mario Equicola, albeit with some variations: 'Hence, it can indeed be said that eyes are the guides in love, especially if they are winsome and soft; black, of a bright and sweet black, or blue; gay and smiling, and in their glance gracious and penetrating like some in whom the channels giving egress to the spirits seem so deep that we can see through them all the way to the heart' (Baldassarre Castiglione,

The Book of the Courtier, edited by D. Javitch (New York: Norton, 2002): 198–199) ('Però ben dir si po che gli occhi siano guida in amore, massimamente se sono graziosi e soavi; neri di quella chiara e dolce negrezza, o vero azzurri; allegri e ridenti e così grati e penetranti nel mirar, come alcuni, nei quali par che quelle vie che danno esito ai spiriti siano tanto profonde, che per esse si vegga insino al core' (Id., *Il libro del Cortegiano* (Turin: Einaudi, 1998): 341)); 'black eyes are praised, and it is said that the goddess of love had such eyes: eyes that are white and black, without marks, broad, sparkling, full, joyful: these are praised by Avicenna, since they demonstrate both wit and the utmost loyalty' ('li occhi se laudano negri, et così dicono haverli havuti la dea della belleza: occhi tra negri et bianchi, senza macula, longhetti, lucidi, tumidetti, alegri: tali sono laudati da Avicenna, per demostrar ingegno et summa fede') (Mario Equicola, *Libro de natura de amore* (Venice: L. Lorio da Portese, 1525): 84r).

xxii. Therefore: *light* is the presence inherent in a luminous source; *illumination* is the physical emanation of light that separates itself from the luminous source; and the *ray* is the means that permits the separation of light in this way. As Aguzzi Barbagli notes (Id., *Un contributo di Francesco Patrizi da Cherso*, 39), this discussion anticipates the deeper exploration of light in the mature work *Nova de universis philosophia*, which appears in the first part entitled *Panaugia*. As Kristeller summarises in relation to the *New Philosophy*: 'Following a well-established earlier usage in Latin, he distinguishes between *lux* and *lumen*. The former is the light as it is found in its source, whereas the latter is the light as it is found diffused outside its source (Bk. I). These two aspects of light are linked with each other by the rays that proceed from the source and pass into surrounding world (Bks. III–IV). In the physical world, light has a special importance as a source of movement and of life' (Kristeller, *Eight Philosophers of the Renaissance*, 119). See also Susana Gómez López, 'Telesio y el debate sobre la naturaleza de la luz en el Renacimiento italiano' in *Telesio y la nueva imagen del mundo en el Renacimiento italiano*, edited by Miguel Á. Granada (Madrid: Siruela, 2013): 194–235.

xxiii. Many of the references in the following discussion (up to D
70) are to Ficino: the luminous nature of the eyes of nocturnal
animals; the experiment of exerting pressure on the eye; the
luminescent eyes of Augustus and Tiberius, as described by
Svetonius; the transmission of disease through the gaze; and
the reference to the blood-stained mirror of the menstruating
woman, derived from Aristotle. See Ficino, *On the Nature
of Love*, (VII-4), 190–191. More generally, one of the fundamental sources for the presence of light within the eyes is
Plato's extensive discussion in the *Timaeus*. In describing the
creation of the human being, and in particular the organs that
will be placed within the head, it is specified precisely why 'the
eyes were the first of the organs to be fashioned by the gods,
to conduct light. The reason why they fastened them within
the head is this. They contrived that such fire as was not for
burning but for providing a gentle light should become a body,
proper to each day. Now the pure fire inside us, cousin to that
fire, they made to flow through the eyes: so they made the
eyes – the eye as a whole but its middle in particular – close-
textured, smooth, and dense, to enable them to keep out all
the other, coarser stuff, and let that kind of fire pass through
pure by itself. Now whenever daylight surrounds the visual
stream, like makes contact with like and coalesces with it to
make up a single homogeneous body aligned with the direction
of the eyes. This happens wherever the internal fire strikes and
presses against an external object it has connected with. And
because this body of fire has become uniform throughout and
thus uniformly affected, it transmits the motions of whatever it
comes in contact with as well as of whatever comes in contact
with it, to and through the whole body until they reach the
soul. This brings about the sensation we call "seeing"' (Plato,
Timaeus, edited by D. J. Zeyl, (Indianapolis: Hackett, 2000),
(45b–d), 33).

xxiv. See Plutarch, *Parallel Lives: Pyrrhus and Marius* (XXXIX).

xxv. Svetonius, *The Twelve Caesars. Tiberius* (III), LXVIII, 2.

xxvi. Svetonius, *The Twelve Caesars. Divus Augustus* (II), LXXIX, 3.

xxvii. Aristotle, *On Dreams*, in Id., *On the Soul. Parva Naturalia.
On Breath*, edited by W. S. Hett (Cambridge (MA) – London:
Harvard University Press – W. Heinemann, 1964), (II, 459b),

357: 'An example of the rapidity with which the sense organs perceive even a slight difference is found in the behaviour of mirrors; a subject which, even considered by itself, would give scope for careful study and investigation. At the same time it is quite clear from this instance that the organ of sight not only is acted upon by its object, but acts reciprocally upon it. If a woman looks into a highly polished mirror during the menstrual period, the surface of the mirror becomes clouded with a blood-red colour (and if the mirror is a new one the stain is not easy to remove, but if it is an old one there is less difficulty). The reason for this is that, as we have said, the organ of sight not only is acted upon by the air, but also sets up an active process, just as bright objects do; for the organ of sight is itself a bright object possessing colour. Now it is reasonable to suppose that at the menstrual periods the eyes are in the same state as any other part of the body; and there is the additional fact that they are naturally full of blood-vessels. Thus when menstruation takes place, as the result of a feverish disorder of the blood, the difference of condition in the eyes, though invisible to us, is none the less real (for the nature of the menses and of the semen is the same); and the eyes set up a movement in the air. This imparts a certain quality to the layer of air extending over the mirror, and assimilates it to itself; and this layer affects the surface of the mirror'.

xxviii. Here Patrizi takes up Ficino's theme of the transmission of disease through the gaze (see the introductory essay, **pp. 15– 16**), though he dilutes the dramatic force of the original discussion. As Aguzzi Barbagli notes (*Un contributo di Francesco Patrizi*, 43), this subject was already present in the classical tradition. An emblematic example is Ovid, *The Cures for Love*, in Id., *The Love Poems*, edited by A. D. Melville (Oxford – New York: Oxford University Press, 1990): (vv. 615–616), 167: 'Eyes that look close at wounds themselves are wounded;/ Infection also injury will do'; see also Plutarch, 'On those who are said to cast an evil eye', in Id., *Quaestiones Convivales* (v-7), in *Plutarch's Moralia, vol 8*, edited by P. A. Clement and H. B. Hoffleit (London – Cambridge (MA): Heinemann – Harvard University Press, 1969): 417–433.

xxix. Petrarch, *The Canzoniere, or Rerum Vulgarium Fragmenta,*
edited by M. Musa (Indianapolis: Indiana University Press,
1999), (233):

'How fortunate for me that from one of
the two loveliest eyes that ever were,
when I saw them disturbed and dark with pain,
there came a force that made mine sick and dim!

To me who had return to break the fast
of seeing her, my sole care in the world,
Heaven and Love have been less harsh than all
the other graces I've received collected;

for from the right eye – better, the right sun –
of my lady to my own right eye there came
the illness that delights me with no pain;

as if it had an intellect and wings,
it transferred like a star shoots through the sky,
Nature and Pity giving it its course'
('Qual ventura mi fu, quando da l'uno
de' duo i piú belli occhi che mai furo,
mirandol di dolor turbato et scuro,
mosse vertú che fe''l mio infermo et bruno!

Send'io tornato a solver il digiuno
di veder lei che sola al mondo curo,
fummi il Ciel e Amor men che mai duro,
se tutte altre mie grazie inseme aduno:

che dal destr'occhio, anzi dal destro sole
de la mia donna al mio destr'occhio venne
il mal che mi diletta, e non mi dole;

e pur com'intelletto avesse e penne,
passò quasi una stella che'n ciel vole;
e Natura e Pietate il corso tenne'.

Petrarca, *Canzoniere*, (Turin: Einaudi, 2011), 379). On the use of a poetic text as a physiological and philosophical source see the introductory essay, **pp. 34–35**. The close connection between poetry, philosophical knowledge and medicinal knowledge is a prominent feature of Ficino's work.

xxx. This theme derives from Ficino, *On the Nature of Love* (VI-6), 123. Ficino nevertheless clearly distinguishes between this reflection on the ideal beauty innate within the soul and his discussion of the contamination of blood.

xxxi. Here Patrizi refers in less dramatic terms to a theme explored by Ficino in much greater depth: the moral *obligation* for reciprocity within permissible love. Ficino, *On the Nature of Love*, (II-8), 30: 'By loving, each surrenders his soul, and by loving in return he restores he other's soul through his own! And so it stands to reason that anyone who is loved should love in return. And anyone who does not love the lover is guilty of murder, or, to be more accurate, he is a thief, a murderer, and a desecrator. Money is possessed by the body, and the body by the soul. And therefore anyone who steals the soul, which possesses both body and money, steals body and money along with the soul, and as a thief, murderer, and desecrator he should be condemned to be put to death three times. As a man of infamy and impiety he can be slain with impunity by anyone if he fails to fulfil the law voluntarily by loving his lover' (*El libro dell'amore*, (II-8), 42: L'uno e l'altro amando dà la sua, e riamando per la sua restituisce l'anima d'altri; per la qual cosa per ragione debba rimanere qualunque è amato, e chi non ama l'amante è in colpa d'omicidio, anzi è ladro, omicidiale e sacrilego. La pecunia dal corpo è posseduta, e'l corpo dall'animo; adunque chi rapisce l'animo dal quale e il corpo e la pecunia si possiede, costui rapisce insieme l'animo, el corpo e la pecunia, il perché come ladro, omicidiale e sacrilego si debba a tre morti condannare, e come infame e impio può sanza pena da ciascuno essere ucciso; se già lui medesimo spontaneamente non adempie la legge, e questo è ch'egli ami l'amante suo'. Here, too, Ficino adapts specific poetic topoi to his philosophical purpose, in this instance from the much-loved tradition of the *dolce stil novo*. It is sufficient to recall the two celebrated *terzine* in which Dante's Francesca, describing the origin of her love for Paolo, summarises several important stilnovist principles: 'Love, which quickly lays hold on gentle heart, seized this one for the fair person that was taken from me, and the mode still hurts me. Love, which absolves no loved one from loving, seized me for the pleasing of him so strongly that, as thou seest, it does not even now abandon me' (Dante, *The Divine Comedy, vol. 1*, (Inf.-5, vv. 100–105), edited by C. Eliot Norton (Boston – New York: Houghton, Mifflin and Company, 1902): 33;

> 'Amor, ch'al cor gentil ratto s'apprende,
> prese costui de la bella persona
> che mi fu tolta; e'l modo ancor m'offende.
> Amor, ch'a nullo amato amar perdona,
> mi prese del costui piacer sì forte,
> che, come vedi, ancor non m'abbandona'

Dante, *Commedia – Inferno* (Milan: Garzanti, 2008): 50–51).

xxxii. Patrizi's attention to anatomical detail reaches a high-water mark in this passage. As Aguzzi Barbagli notes (*Un contributo di Francesco Patrizi*, 46), this conception of the *spiritus* as originating from the heart, its connection with blood and fusion with the air during cardiac expansion and contraction (which today we term *systole* and *diastole*) lacks the more metaphysical implications of Plato and Ficino, yet is nevertheless present in Vesalius, demonstrating its significance in contemporary medicine. It is therefore interesting encounter this passage in Patrizi, but also Ficino's discussion of the *spiritus* observed above (see Ficino, *Three Books on Life*, (I-2), 111), with which Vesalius concurs: 'Quemadmodum itaque cordis substantiæ, vitalis animæ vis, ac propriæ iecoris carni, naturalis animæ facultas induntur, insuper ut iecur crassiorem sanguinem, ac qui perquam caliginosus est, naturalem spiritum, et cor item rursus sanguinem impetu per corpus ruentem una cum vitali spiritu conficiunt, et perinde atque hæc viscera per dedicatos sibi canales omnibus corporis partibus suas materias derivant, ita quoque cerebrum aptam ipsius muneri obtinens materiam, in proprijs sedibus, ac illius functioni apposite subministrantibus instrumentis, animalem spiritum longe clarissimum tenuissimumque parat, quo ad divinas principis animæ operationes partim utitur, partim autem ad sensuum motusque instrumenta per nervos tanquam per funiculos continuo distribuit, ea nunquam spiritu, qui præcipuus eorum instrumentorum functionis autor censetur' (Andreas Vesalius, *De humani corporis fabrica. Libri Septem* (VII-1) (Basel: J. Oporinus, 1543): 622). Vesalius had earlier stated that 'nihilominus interim de animæ facultatibus, functionibus, substantia, natura, speciebus, et earum sedibus investigatione remissa, libere asseremus cor facultatis, atque adeo spiritus vitalis fontem, et caloris nativi sedem fomitemque existere, ac pulsuum autorem essem, singulasque cordis partes illi ad calorem spiritumque spectanti usui subservire commonstrabimus' (*ivi* (VI-15), 594–5); and a few pages later "quemadmodum enim dexter [ventriculus cordis] ex cava sanguinem trahit, ita quoque sinister aerem ex pulmone in arteriam venalem attractum, ad se dilatato corde allicit, illosque ad caloris innati refrigerationem et substantiæ ipsius enutritione, spiritumque vitalem utitur, hunc aerem excoquens et præparans, ut is una cum sanguine qui ex dextro ventriculo in sinistrum per ventriculorum septum copiosius resudavit in magnam arteriam, totumque adeo corpus delegari possit" (ibid. (vi-15), 598); see Fig. 1.3.

xxxiii. The discussion now turns back towards the question that began the dialogue: the pleasure associated with the kiss.

xxxiv. Here we move into the final section of the work, in which the various categories of the kiss are examined in light of the philosophical and physiological theories discussed up to this point.

xxxv. This discussion echoes Ficino, who explores the rage and desire for revenge typical of the madness caused by the amorous disease (see Ficino, *On the Nature of Love*, (VII-5), 143–144; *El libro dell'amore*, VII-5, 196–197). Here, the question is radically reinterpreted in terms of an erotic game. The theme of the love as death, understood in a positive sense as that from which a new life is derived, is nevertheless also present in Ficino, where it is obviously discussed in relation to love that is permissible and therefore without the overtone of revenge inherent in the amorous disease. Ficino states that 'something amazing happens when two love each other: A lives in B, and B lives in A. They make an exchange, in which each gives himself to the other, in order to receive the other. [...] It is rather that each possesses himself and the other, for A possesses himself, but in

B. There is no that while I love you, who love me, I re-discover myself in you, who are thinking of me. And I re-gain myself, who am spurned by myself, in you, who are looking after me. You do the same in me. There is something else that strikes me as amazing: if, after losing myself, I re-gain myself through you, then I possess myself through you. If I possess myself through you, I possess you first, and I possess you more than I possess myself; and I am closer to you than I am to myself, for I approach myself through no means other than yourself. In this respect the power of Cupid is different from the might of Mars, because imperial rule and Love are different in this way. It is through himself that the ruler possesses others; it is through another than the lover re-gains himself [...] In reciprocal Love there is only a single death, but a double resurrection, because the lover dies once in himself when he abandons himself, but he is at once brought back to life in his beloved when his beloved welcomes him back with warm thoughts, and he is brought back to life a second time when he eventually recognises himself in his beloved and has no doubt that he is loved in return. What a blessed death, being followed by two lives! What a marvellous agreement, in which a man gives himself for another and possesses the other without losing himself! What an incalculable gain, when two become one in such a way that each of the two becomes two for a single one!' (*On the Nature of Love*, (II-8), 29–30) (*El libro dell'amore*, (II-8), 41–42: 'cosa maravigliosa adviene quando due insieme s'amano: costui in colui e colui in costui vive. Costoro fanno a cambio insieme e ciascuno dà sé ad altri per altri ricevere. [...] Anzi l'uno e l'altro ha sé medesimo, e ha altrui, perché questo ha sé ma in colui, colui possiede sé ma in costui. Certamente mentre che io amo te amante me, io in te cogitante di me ritruovo me, e me da me medesimo sprezzato in te conservante racquisto; quel medesimo in me tu fai. Questo ancora mi pare meraviglioso: imperò che io, da poi che me medesimo perdetti, se per te mi racquisto, per te ho me. Se per te io ho me, io ho te prima e più anche me, e sono più ad te che a me propinquo, con ciò sia che io non m'accosto a me per altro mezzo che per te. In questo la virtù di Cupidine dalla forza di Marte è differente: perché lo imperio e l'amore sono così differenti. Lo'mperadore per sé altri possiede, l'amatore per altri ripiglia sé [...]. Una solamente è la morte nell'amore reciproco, le resurrezioni sono due; perché chi ama muore una volta in sé quando si lascia, risuscita subito nello amato quando l'amato lo riceve con ardente pensiero, risuscita ancora quando lui nello amato finalmente si riconosce e non dubita sé essere amato. O felice morte alla quale seguitano due vite! O maraviglioso contracto nel quale l'uomo dà sé per altri, e ha altri, e sé non lascia! O inestimabile guadagno quando due in tal modo uno divengono, che ciascheduno de' dua per uno solo diventa due').

xxxvi. As Gómez López observes (*La fisiología del amor*, 49), the solution to this unresolved question is most likely found in the suggestion that the kiss on the left side of the neck produces the most pleasure, which recalls the physiology of Galen. According to Galen's model, *natural spirits* are generated in the liver and some of them travel with the blood to the right ventricle of the heart via the vena cava. Part of this blood follows the arterial vein to the lungs, while the remainder passes through the septum to the left ventricle. Here the venous blood mixes with air coming from the lungs (*pneuma*), becoming arterial and generating *vital spirits*. The left part of the neck is closer to this area, and thus permits greater absorption of *spiritus* directly from the heart.

xxxvii. The idea of the eyes as both the origin and cure of the wound of love is also present in Ficino, where it is related to the amorous disease. While for Patrizi the wound is broadly metaphorical but the antidote is real, in Ficino the opposite is the case. Having been virulently wounded by the ocular rays of the beloved, the lover continuously searches for them, not because they represent a true antidote but because of self-destructive dependency: 'But the case [of the evil eye] is very serious when the younger person wounds the heart of the older person. This, my dear friends, is what Apuleius complains of when he says, "You alone are the whole cause and origin of my grief, and at the same time you are my medicine and well-being. For these eyes of yours, passing through mine into the very centre of my heart, ignite a fierce fire in my very marrow. Have mercy, therefore, on him who is dying on account of you"' (*On the Nature of Love*, VII-4, 141; *El libro dell'amore*,

(VII-4), 193: 'Ma quello è mal d'occhio gravissimo, nel quale la persona più giovane el cuore della più vecchia ferisce; questo è quello, amici miei, di che el platonico Apuleio si rammalica così dicendo: «La cagione tutta e l'origine di questo mio dolore, e ancora la medicina e la salute mia, se' tu solo, perché questi tuoi occhi per questi mia occhi passando infino al centro del mio cuore, uno acerrimo incendio nelle midolle mie commuovono. Adunque abbi misericordia di costui el quale per tua cagione perisce»'). The source Ficino is referring to is Apuleius, *Metamorphoses* (X, III-20).

xxxviii. In this sequence Patrizi reveals first why the lover is compelled, more or less consciously, to kiss the various parts of the beloved's body, and next the reasons that determine the differing degree of pleasure (see the table of kisses in the introductory essay, **p. 30**). While the types of kisses corresponding to the parts of the body are listed, the various methods of kissing (with the exception of the biting kiss) are not. The author likely judged that these could be straightforwardly deduced from the theory he has delineated, with no need for further explication.

xxxix. It is significant that the work concludes with a poetic composition that retraces its essential points, serving as a kind of summary. On the relationship between poetry, philosophical knowledge and medical knowledge, which we have already discussed, see the introductory essay (**pp. 34–35, 42–43**).

Bibliography

Selection of Patrizi's Works

Patrizi F., 'A Baccio Valori. Firenze 1587' in *Lettere ed opuscoli inediti.*

Patrizi F., *Della Historia. Diece dialoghi di M. Francesco Patritio ne'quali si ragiona di tutte le cose appartenenti all'historia, e allo scriverla, e all'osservarla* (Venice: A. Arrivabene, 1560).

Patrizi F., 'Discorso di M. Francesco Patritio,' in Luca Contile, *Le rime di Messer Luca Contile, divise in tre parti, con discorsi, et argomenti di M. Francesco Patritio, et M. Antonio Borghesi. Nuovamente stampate. Con le sei Canzoni dette le* Sei Sorelle di Marte (Venice: F. Sansovino, 1560): 14r–25v.

Patrizi F., *Du baiser*, edited by Sylvie Laurens Aubry (Paris: Les Belles Lettres, 2002).

Patrizi F., 'Il Delfino overo del Bacio' in *Lettere ed opuscoli inediti*, edited by Danilo Aguzzi Barbagli (Florence: Istituto Nazionale di Studi sul Rinascimento, 1975): 135–164.

Patrizi F., 'La città felice' in Id., *La città felice. Dialogo dell'honore, il Barignano. Discorso della diversità de' furori poetici. Lettura sopra il sonetto del Petrarca.* La gola, e'l sonno e l'ociose piume (Venice: G. Griffio, 1553).

Patrizi F., 'Lettura sopra il sonetto del Petrarca. *La gola, e'l sonno e l'ociose piume*', in *La città felice. Dialogo dell'honore, il Barignano. Discorso della diversità de' furori poetici. Lettura sopra il sonetto del Petrarca.* La gola, e'l sonno e l'ociose piume.

Patrizi F., *L'amorosa filosofia*, edited by John C. Nelson (Florence: Le Monnier, 1963).

T. Ghezzani, *The 'Kiss' and the Medicine of Love*,
Palgrave Studies in Medieval and Early Modern Medicine,
https://doi.org/10.1007/978-3-031-75283-4

Patrizi F., *Nova de universis philosophia, in qua aristotelica methodo non per motum sed per lucem, et lumina, ad primam causam ascenditur. Deinde propria Patricii methodo, tota in contemplationem venit Divinitas. Postremo methodo Platonica, rerum universitas, a conditore Deo deducitur* (Ferrara: B. Mammarelli, 1591).

Patrizi F., *The Philosophy of Love*, edited by D. Pastina and J. W. Crayton (Philadelphia: Xlibris, 2003).

SELECTION OF WORKS RELEVANT TO THE DIALOGUE

Aristotle, *On Dreams*, in Id., *On the Soul. Parva Naturalia. On Breath*, edited by W. S. Hett (Cambridge (MA) – London: Harvard University Press – W. Heinemann, 1964).

Bembo P., *Gli Asolani* (Bloomington: Indiana University Press, 1954).

Bembo P., *Gli Asolani* (Florence: Accademia della Crusca, 1991).

Castiglione B., *Il libro del Cortegiano* (Turin: Einaudi, 1998).

Castiglione B., *The Book of the Courtier*, edited by D. Javitch (New York: Norton, 2002).

Contile L., 'A M. Franc. Patricio. 1562' in Id., *Il secondo volume delle Lettere di Luca Contile*, (G. Bartoli: Venice, 1564): 150v.

Dante, *Commedia – Inferno* (Milan: Garzanti, 2008).

Dante, *The Divine Comedy, vol. 1*, edited by C. Eliot Norton (Boston – New York: Houghton, Mifflin and Company, 1902).

Equicola M., *Libro de natura de amore* (Venice: L. Lorio da Portese, 1525).

Ficino M., 'Commentaria in Platonis "Sophistam"' in *Icastes. Marsilio Ficino's Interpretation of Plato's Sophist*, edited by Michael J. B. Allen (Berkeley: University of California Press, 1989).

Ficino M., *El libro dell'amore* (Florence: Olschki, 1987).

Ficino M., *On the Nature of Love: Ficino on Plato's Symposium* (London: Shepheard – Walwyn, 2016).

Ficino M., *Three Books on Life* (Arizona: Medieval & Renaissance Texts & Studies – The Renaissance Society of America, 1998).

Nifo A., *De pulchro et amore* (Rome: A. Blado, 1529).

Ovid, *The Cures for Love*, in Id., *The Love Poems*, edited by A. D. Melville (Oxford – New York: Oxford University Press, 1990).

Petrarca, *Canzoniere* (Turin: Einaudi, 2011).

Petrarca, *The Canzoniere, or Rerum Vulgarium Fragmenta*, edited by M. Musa (Indianapolis: Indiana University Press, 1999).

Pico della Mirandola G., 'Commento sopra una canzona de amore composta da Girolamo Benivieni' in Id., *De hominis dignitate, Heptaplus, De ente et uno, e scritti vari* (Florence: Vallecchi, 1942): 443–581.

Plato, *Gorgias*, edited by W. Hamilton (Baltimore – Maryland: Penguin, 1960).

Plato, *Phaedrus*, edited by R. Hackforth (Cambridge: Cambridge University Press, 1997).

Plato, *Symposium*, edited by A. Sharon (Newburyport: Focus Publishing, 1998).

Plato, *Timaeus*, edited by D. J. Zeyl (Indianapolis: Hackett, 2000).

Plutarch, *Moralia, vol. 8*, edited by P. A. Clement and H. B. Hoffleit (London – Cambridge (MA): Heinemann – Harvard University Press, 1969).

Secundus J., *Basia* in Id., *The Love Poems* (London: G. Routledge, 1930).

Vesalius A., *De humani corporis fabrica. Libri Septem* (Basel: J. Oporinus, 1543).

SELECTION OF STUDIES ON PATRIZI

Aguzzi Barbagli D., 'Un contributo di Francesco Patrizi da Cherso alle dottrine rinascimentali sull'amore,' *Yearbook of Italian Studies*, 2 (1972): 19–50.

Akopyan O., 'Francesco Patrizi da Cherso (1529–1597): new perspectives on a Renaissance philosopher,' *Intellectual History Review*, 29 (2019): 541–543.

Banić-Pajnić E., 'Marsilio Ficino and Franciscus Patricius on Love' in *Francesco Patrizi. Philosopher of the Renaissance*, edited by Tomáš Nejeschleba and Paul R. Blum (Olomouc: Centre for Renaissance Texts, 2014): 213–231.

Bolzoni L., 'A proposito di una recente edizione di inediti patriziani,' *Rinascimento*, 16 (1976): 133–156.

Bolzoni L., *L'universo dei poemi possibili. Studi su Francesco Patrizi da Cherso* (Rome: Bulzoni, 1980).

Borsetto L., '«Concetti da porre in amorosa poesia». L'*accessus* neoplatonico del Patrizi alle Rime di Luca Contile' in Ead., *Riscrivere gli Antichi, riscrivere i Moderni e altri studi di letteratura italiana e comparata tra Quattro e Ottocento* (Alessandria: Edizioni dell'Orso, 2002): 303–320.

Bottin F., 'Francesco Patrizi e l'aristotelismo padovano,' *Quaderni per la storia dell'Università di Padova*, 32 (1999): 163–176.

Castelli P. (edited by), *Francesco Patrizi. Filosofo platonico nel crepuscolo del Rinascimento* (Florence: Olschki, 2002).

Ghezzani T., *Il Platonico innamorato. Poesia, Amore, Magia in Francesco Patrizi da Cherso* (Florence: Olschki, 2023).

Ghezzani T., 'Medicamenti della memoria e medicamenti dell'anima: *ferita amorosa e carnalità* tra Marsilio Ficino e Francesco Patrizi,' *Bruniana & Campanelliana*, 29 (2023).

Gómez López S., 'La fisiología del amor. El diálogo de Francesco Patrizi sobre los besos,' *Prometeica. Revista de Filosofía y Ciencias*, 24 (2022): 32–54.

Gómez López S., 'Medicina y política en Francesco Patrizi: el cuerpo de *La ciudad feliz*,' *Asclepio. Revista de Historia de la Ciencia y de la Medicina*, 61 (2015): 1–14.

Kristeller P. O., *Eight Philosophers of the Italian Renaissance* (Stanford-California: Stanford University Press, 1964).

Morosini R., 'Patrizi da Cherso: How and why neoplatonic kisses can give pleasure,' *Accademia. Révue de la Société Marsile Ficin*, 24 (2022): 69–84.

Muccillo M., 'Dall'ordine dei libri all'ordine della realtà: ordine e metodo nella filosofia di Francesco Patrizi' in *Francesco Patrizi. Philosopher of the Renaissance*, 9–61.

Muccillo M., 'La dissoluzione del paradigma aristotelico' in *Le filosofie del Rinascimento*, edited by Cesare Vasoli (Milan: B. Mondadori, 2002): 506–533.

Muccillo M., 'Marsilio Ficino e Francesco Patrizi da Cherso' in *Marsilio Ficino e il ritorno di Platone. Studi e documenti*, vol. 2, edited by Gian Carlo Garfagnini (Florence: Olschki 1986): 615–679.

Muccillo M., 'Philosophy and Orthodoxy: Valuation and Devaluation of the Platonic Tradition in the Late Renaissance' in *Transforming Topoi: The Exigencies and Impositions of Tradition*, edited by A. J. Johnston et al. (Göttingen: V&R, 2018): 89–118.

Nelson J. C., '«L'amorosa filosofia» di Francesco Patrizi da Cherso,' *Rinascimento*, 2 (1962): 89–106.

Palumbo M., 'Patrizi, Francesco' in *Dizionario biografico degli italiani, vol. 81* (Rome: Istituto dell'Enciclopedia italiana, 2014).

Pietrobon E., 'Gli *Argomenti* di Francesco Patrizi come teatro ermeneutico del testo' in *Canzonieri in transito. Lasciti petrarcheschi e nuovi archetipi letterari tra Cinque e Seicento*, edited by Alessandro Metlica and Franco Tomasi (Milan-Udine: Mimesis, 2015): 37–58.

Plastina S., 'La figura e l'opera di Francesco Patrizi da Cherso nella critica più recente,' *Bruniana & Campanelliana*, 3 (1997): 335–344.

Prins J., *Echoes of an Invisible World. Marsilio Ficino and Francesco Patrizi on Cosmic Order and Music Theory* (Leiden-Boston: Brill, 2014).

Puliafito A. L., 'La fisica telesiana attraverso gli occhi di un contemporaneo: Francesco Patrizi da Cherso' in *Bernardino Telesio e la cultura napoletana*, edited by Raffaelle Sirri and Maurizio Torrini (Naples: Guida, 1992): 257–270.

Scapparone E., 'Patrizi, Francesco' in *Il Contributo italiano alla storia del Pensiero – Filosofia* (Rome: Istituto dell'Enciclopedia Italiana, 2012).

Škamperle I., '*L'amorosa filosofia* di Frane Petrić e il concetto di *Philautia*,' *Prilozi*, 75 (2012): 23–34.

Vasoli C., 'Il «Proemio» di Francesco Patrizi alla *Nova de universis philosophia*' in *I margini del libro. Indagine teorica e storica sui testi di dedica*, edited by Maria Antonietta Terzoli (Rome-Padua: Antenore, 2004): 77–115.

Vasoli C., '«L'amorosa filosofia»: dall'«amore platonico» all'universale «philautia»' in Id., *Francesco Patrizi da Cherso* (Rome: Bulzoni, 1989): 181–204.

Vasoli C., 'Un filosofo tra lo Studio e la Corte: Patrizi a Ferrara' in *Francesco Patrizi da Cherso*: 205–228.

Vuilleumier Laurens F., 'Les Basia de Jean Second et la tradition philosophique de Marsile Ficin à Francesco Patrizi' in *La poétique de Jean Second et son influence au xvie siècle*, edited by Jean Balsamo and Pettine Galand-Hallyn (Paris: Les Belles Lettres, 2000): 25–38.

SELECTION OF STUDIES RELEVANT TO THE CONTEXT OF THE DIALOGUE

Benassi S., 'Marsilio Ficino e il potere dell'immaginazione,' *I castelli di Yale*, 2 (1997): 1–18.

Bolzoni L., *The Gallery of Memory. Literary and Iconographic Models in the Age of the Printing Press* (Toronto – Buffalo – London: University of Toronto Press, 2001).

Brown A., *The Return of Lucretius to Renaissance Florence* (Cambridge (MA.)- London: Harvard University Press, 2010).

Burckhardt J., *The Civilization of the Renaissance in Italy* (Vienna: Phaidon Press, 1954).

Busi G. and Ebgi R. (edited by), *Giovanni Pico della Mirandola. Mito, magia, qabbalah* (Turin: Einaudi, 2014).

Canone E., 'Il «senso» nei trattati d'amore: Ficino e la fortuna del modello platonico nel Cinquecento' in *Sensus-Sensatio. VIII Colloquio internazionale del Lessico Intellettuale Europeo*, edited by Massimo L. Bianchi (Florence: Olschki, 1996): 177–198.

Ciavolella M., 'Eros e Memoria nella cultura del Rinascimento' in *La cultura della memoria*, edited by Lina Bolzoni and Pietro Corsi (Bologna: Il Mulino, 1992): 319–333.

Ciavolella, M. 'Eros/Ereos? Marsio Ficino's Interpretation of Guido Cavalcanti's "Donna me prega"' in *Ficino and Renaissance Neoplatonism*, edited by Konrad Eisenbichler and Olga Zorzi Pugliese (Ottawa: Dovehouse, 1986): 39–48.

Ciavolella M., *La "malattia d'amore" dall'Antichità al Medioevo* (Rome: Bulzoni, 1976).

Corrias A., 'Imagination and Memory in Marsilio Ficino's Theory of the Vehicles of the Soul,' *The International Journal of the Platonic Tradition*, 6 (2012): 81–114.

Couliano I. P., *Eros and Magic in the Renaissance* (Chicago – London: University of Chicago Press, 1987).

Dolfin B. G., *I Dolfin (Delfino) patrizii veneziani nella storia di Venezia dall'anno 452 al 1923* (Milan: F. Parenti, 1924).

Ebgi R., *Voluptas. La filosofia del piacere nel giovane Marsilio Ficino (1457–1469)* (Pisa: Edizioni della Normale – Istituto Nazionale di Studi sul Rinascimento, 2019).

Ernst G. and Giglioni G. (edited by), *I vincoli della natura. Magia e stregoneria nel Rinascimento* (Rome: Carocci, 2012).

Fellina S., *Modelli di episteme neoplatonica nella Firenze del '400: le gnoseologie di Giovanni Pico della Mirandola e di Marsilio Ficino* (Florence: Olschki, 2014).

Ferretto S., *Maestri per il metodo di trattar le cose. Bassiano Lando, Giovanni Battista da Monte e la scienza della medicina nel XVI secolo* (Padua: CLEUP, 2012).

Garin E., *Ermetismo del Rinascimento* (Pisa: Edizioni della Normale, 2006);

Garin E., 'La filosofia dell'amore. Sincretismo platonico-aristotelico' in Id., *Storia della filosofia italiana, vol.* 2 (Turin: Einaudi, 1966): 581–615.

Garin E., '*Phantasia* e *Imaginatio* fra Marsilio Ficino e Pietro Pomponazzi' in *Phantasia-Imaginatio. V Colloquio internazionale del Lessico Intellettuale Europeo* edited by Marta Fattori and Massimo L. Bianchi (Rome: Edizioni dell'Ateneo, 1988): 3–20.

Garin E., 'Relazione introduttiva' in *Spiritus. IV Colloquio internazionale del Lessico Intellettuale Europeo*, edited by Marta Fattori and Massimo L. Bianchi (Roma: Edizioni dell'Ateneo, 1984): 3–14.

Gentile S., '*Commentarium in Convivium de amore / El libro dell'Amore* di Marsilio Ficino' in *Letteratura italiana. Le opere, vol.* 2, edited by Alberto Asor Rosa (Milan: Einaudi, 1992): 743–767.

Gentile S., 'Ficino, Epicuro e Lucrezio' in *The Rebirth of Platonic Theology. Proceedings of a conference held at The Harvard University Center for Italian Renaissance Studies (Villa I Tatti) and the Istituto Nazionale di Studi sul Rinascimento (Florence, 26–27 April 2007)*, edited by James Hankins and Fabrizio Meroi (Florence: Olschki, 2013): 119–135.

Ghezzani T., 'Immagini della *servitù volontaria* tra Marsilio Ficino e Giovanni Pico della Mirandola. Problemi di filosofia d'amore,' *Philosophia. Rivista della Società Italiana di Storia della Filosofia*, 1 (2019): 65–91.

Giglioni G., 'Contagio e immaginazione,' *Lexicon philosophicum*, 8 (2020): 265–268.

Giovannozzi D., '«Filosofando e vagando per lo gran mare della sua essenzia». Testi e temi della trattatistica d'amore nel Rinascimento,' *Bruniana & Campanelliana*, 27 (2021): 327–333.

Gómez López S., 'Telesio y el debate sobre la naturaleza de la luz en el Renacimiento italiano' in *Telesio y la nueva imagen del mundo en el Renacimiento italiano*, edited by Miguel Á. Granada (Madrid: Siruela, 2013): 194–235.

Guarna V., *L'Accademia Veneziana della Fama (1557–1561). Storia, cultura e editoria. Con l'edizione della* Somma delle opere *(1558) e altri documenti inediti* (Rome: Vecchiarelli, 2018).

Gurashi D., *In deifico speculo. Agrippa's humanism* (Paderborn: Brill-Fink, 2021).

Hankins J., 'The Invention of the Platonic Academy in Florence,' *Rinascimento*, 41 (2001): 3–38.

Klein R., *Form and Meaning. Essays on the Renaissance and Modern Art* (New York: Viking Press, 1979).

Klibansky R., Panofsky E., Saxl F., *Saturn and Melancholy. Studies in the History of Natural Philosophy, Religion and Art* (Nendeln – Liechtenstein: Kraus Reprint, 1979).

Kristeller P. O., *Iter Italicum, vol. 1* (London – Leiden: Brill, 1963).

Kristeller P. O., *The Philosophy of Marsilio Ficino* (Gloucester: P. Smith, 1964).

Lazzarin F., 'L'ideale del *severe ludere* nel pensiero di Marsilio Ficino,' *Accademia. Révue de la Société Marsile Ficin*, 7 (2005): 61–79.

Lazzarin F., 'Poesia e filosofia in Marsilio Ficino' in *Para/Textuelle Verhandlungen zwischen Dichtung und Philosophie in der Frühen Neuzeit*, edited by Bernhard Huss et al. (Berlin-New York: De Gruyter, 2011): 229–247.

Leitgeb M. C., *Amore e magia. La nascita di Eros e il De amore di Ficino* (Lucca: Cahiers Accademia, 2006).

Maggi A., 'La fase conclusiva dei trattati d'amore rinascimentali nell'autocommento poetico di Tasso' in *Indagini su Tasso. Atti del convengo internazionale. Sorrento, 6-8 novembre 2017*, edited by Alfonso Paolella (Naples: Eidos, 2018): 117–136.

Molinarolo F., 'Lo spettro della fantasia: teoria dell'anima, etica e apologetica nel *De Imaginatione* di Gianfrancesco Pico della Mirandola' in Giovanni Francesco Pico della Mirandola, *L'immaginazione* (Pisa: Edizioni della Normale – Istituto Nazionale di Studi sul Rinascimento, 2022): 7–168.

Nardi B., 'L'amore e i medici medievali' in Id., *Saggi e note di critica dantesca* (Milan-Naples: Ricciardi, 1966): 238–267.

Nelson J. C., *Theory of Love: The Context of Giordano Bruno's "Eroici Furori"* (New York: Columbia University Press, 1958).

Nicoli E., 'Ficino, Lucretius and Atomism,' *Early Science and Medicine*, 23 (2018): 330–361.

Palmer A., *Reading Lucretius in the Renaissance* (Cambridge (MA.)-London: Harvard University Press, 2014).

Panichi N., 'Introduction' in Michel de Montaigne, *De la force de l'imagination. Essais, I, 21* (Paris: Classiques Garnier, 2021): 11–61.

Perella N. J., *The Kiss Sacred and Profane: An Interpretative History of Kiss Simbolysme and Related Religio-Erotic Themes* (Berkeley-Los Angeles: University of California Press, 1969).

Piro F., *Il retore interno. Immaginazione e passioni all'alba della età moderna* (Naples: La Città del Sole, 1999).

Pozzi M., 'Introduzione' in *Trattati d'Amore del '500*, edited by Id. (Rome-Bari: Laterza, 1975): v–xl.

Prosperi V., *«Di soavi licor gli orli del vaso»*. *La fortuna di Lucrezio dall'U-manesimo alla Controriforma* (Turin: Aragno, 2004).

Rivolta A., *Catalogo dei codici pinelliani dell'Ambrosiana* (Tipografia Pontificia Arcivescovile S. Giuseppe: Milan, 1933).

Sassi M. M., 'The Greek Philosophers on How to Memorise—And Learn' in *Greek Memories. Theories and Practices*, edited by Luca Castagnoli and Paola Ceccarelli (Cambridge: Cambridge University Press, 2019): 343–361.

Tirinnanzi N., *Umbra naturae. L'immaginazione da Ficino a Bruno* (Rome: Edizioni di Storia e Letteratura, 2000).

Torre A., *Scritture ferite. Innesti, doppiaggi e correzioni nella letteratura rinascimentale* (Venice: Marsilio, 2019).

Vanhaelen M., 'Cosmic Harmony, Demons, and the Mnemonic Power of Music in Renaissance Florence. The Case of Marsilio Ficino' in *Sing Aloud Harmonious Spheres. Renaissance Conceptions of Cosmic Harmony*, edited by Jacomien Prins and Maude Vanhaelen (New York: Routledge, 2017).

Vasoli C., 'Le Accademie fra Cinquecento e Seicento e il loro ruolo nella storia della tradizione enciclopedica' in Id., *Immagini umanistiche* (Naples: Morano, 1983): 429–465.

Vernant J. P., *Myth and Thought Among the Greeks* (London – Bonston – Melbourne – Henley: Routledge & Kegan, 1983).

Walker D. P., 'Medical Spirits and God and the Soul' in *Spiritus*: 218–243.

Walker D. P., *Spiritual and Demonic Magic. From Ficino to Campanella* (Notre Dame: University of Notre Dame Press, 1975)

Walker D. P., 'The Astral Body in Renaissance Medicine,' *Journal of the Warburg and Courtald Institutes*, 21 (1958): 119–133.

Yates F. A., *Giordano Bruno and the Hermetic Tradition* (Chicago: University of Chicago Press, 1964).

Yates F. A., *The Art of Memory* (Chicago: The University of Chicago Press, 1966).

Zorzi Pugliese O., 'Variations on Ficino's *De Amore*: The Hymns to Love by Benivieni and Castiglione' in *Ficino and Renaissance Neoplatonism*: 113–121.

INDEX

The manufacturer's authorised representative in the EU is Springer Nature Customer Service Centre GmbH, Europaplatz 3, 69115 Heidelberg, Germany. If you have any concerns regarding our products, please contact ProductSafety@springernature.com

Printed and bound by CPI Group (UK) Ltd, Croydon, CR0 4YY
27/04/2026
02097570-0008